IVF CHILDREN

THE FIRST GENERATION

ASSISTED REPRODUCTION AND CHILD DEVELOPMENT

IVF CHILDREN

THE FIRST GENERATION

ASSISTED REPRODUCTION AND CHILD DEVELOPMENT

Alastair G. Sutcliffe, MD, MRCP, FRCPCH
Senior Lecturer in Paediatrics
University College London

The Parthenon Publishing Group
International Publishers in Medicine, Science & Technology

A CRC PRESS COMPANY
BOCA RATON LONDON NEW YORK WASHINGTON, D.C.

Published in the UK and Europe by
The Parthenon Publishing Group
23–25 Blades Court
Deodar Road
London SW15 2NU, UK

Published in the USA by
The Parthenon Publishing Group
345 Park Avenue South, 10th Floor
New York, NY 10010, USA

British Library Cataloguing-in-Publication Data
Sutcliffe, Alastair G.
IVF Children : the first generation : assisted reproduction and child development
1. Fertilization in vitro, Human 2. Child development
I. Title
618.1 ′ 78059

ISBN 1842141236

Library of Congress Cataloging-in-Publication Data
Data available on request

First published 2002

Typeset by Siva Math Setters, Chennai, India
Printed and bound by Butler & Tanner Ltd., Frome and London, UK

Contents

Dedication

This book is dedicated to my wife Nurhan.

Also to my children Papatya Estella, Jan Bruce and Elâ Iona, all of whom have taught me a lot about child development.

They have kindly given up their Daddy occasionally, to allow me to travel to pursue further studies into the outcomes of assisted reproductive therapies.

Acknowledgements

First, I would like to thank my mentors during my academic and clinical training: Dr Bulugahapitiya, who showed me how to be a good general pediatrician; Dr D'Souza, who introduced me to studies in assisted reproduction outcome and was an excellent mentor during my first project; and Professor Taylor, who supervised my thesis and has been an inspiring leader during my time working for and with him.

I would like to thank all the families who have participated in my research projects, allowing me to share a little of their lives.

Also those colleagues working in reproductive medicine (in the UK, Europe, USA and Australia), both in the clinical setting and in the laboratory, who have through their help allowed me to overcome considerable hurdles to recruit and assess in their clinics children conceived after IVF.

Finally, I would like to thank all those who have contributed to the costs of my research and who are acknowledged in my recent research papers.

1

A brief overview of the development of *in vitro* fertilization, including reference to recent developments

'The greatest danger arises from ruthless application of partial knowledge on a vast scale.'

E.F. Schumacher

INTRODUCTION

Historical overview

The concept of extracorporeal or novel forms of conception has existed for many thousands of years. The ancient Greek legends include many references to unusual conception. The Olympian god Zeus fathered many children with mortal women, often whilst appearing in unusual form. For example, he appeared as a shower of gold to Danae and fathered Perseus; Leda he loved whilst in the shape of a swan and she bore two eggs, one containing the children of Zeus (Pollux and Helen), and the other the children of her husband Tyndareus (Castor and Clytemnestra); Alcmene, wife of Amphitryon, who bore him Heracles; and Europa, whom he abducted in the shape of a white bull and who bore him Minos, Rhadamanthus and Sarpedon.

Jesus Christ was referred to in several places in the Bible as being conceived in a novel way between Mary and the Holy Spirit.

> 'In the sixth month, God sent the angel Gabriel to Nazareth, a town in Galilee to a virgin pledged to be married to a man named Joseph, a descendent of

> David. The virgin's name was Mary ... the angel answered, "The Holy Spirit will come upon you and the power of the Most High will overshadow you. So the holy one to be born will be called the Son of God."'
>
> New International Version of the Bible, Luke 1:26–35

The Bible also provides insight into how the pain of infertility, the driving force behind the need for *in vitro* fertilization (IVF), was perceived on a human level in those times.

> 'When Rachel saw that she was not bearing Jacob any children, she became jealous of her sister. So she said to Jacob, "Give me children, or I'll die!"'
>
> New International Version of the Bible, Genesis 30:1

It was not until 1878 that the first attempts at IVF of mammalian eggs were made. These were by the Viennese embryologist Schenk[1]. Subsequently many attempts were made to fertilize mammalian eggs. Although many successes were claimed, skepticism surrounded the claims of actual fertilization *in vitro*. Schenk, working with rabbit and guinea-pig ova, noted the formation of the second polar body and cell division in culture (after the addition of sperm). He stated that the eggs had developed *in vitro* up to the eight-cell stage.

The pioneering work of Walter Heap[2] in 1891 demonstrated that fertilized eggs from the rabbit could be retrieved and subsequently transferred to a recipient. In 1880 Onanoff[3] reported that rabbit and guinea pig ova taken from the uterus could be fertilized *in vitro* and these subsequently developed when cultured or implanted into the abdominal cavity of females or males of the same or different species. However, it is now thought more likely that Onanoff's ova were fertilized *in vivo*. In 1930, Pincus[4] started work on IVF and embryo transfer in rabbits. He observed sperm penetration in harvested tubal rabbit eggs inseminated *in vitro*. In collaboration with Enzmann[5] he reported the first successful fertilization of mammalian eggs *in vitro* with subsequent birth.

Pioneering work by Pincus and Enzmann[5] in 1935 and 1936 laid the foundations for the understanding of the stages of oocyte maturation and fertilization in mammalian eggs. Pincus and Saunders[6] later extended these studies to human oocytes (further defining the maturation process of human ova).

In the USA, Rock and colleagues[7] used the work of Ogino (which led to the rhythm method of family planning) to establish the time of ovulation using laparoscopy. Using similar methods, Pincus and Hertig attempted to recover ovulated human ova from Fallopian tubes removed at surgery. Lewis and Gregory[8] obtained cinematographic views of rabbit eggs developing from the one- to the eight-cell stage. Over a 20-year period from the beginning of this work, an enormous bank of information on early human embryos was established. In 1935 Menkin and Rock[9] claimed that they had successfully fertilized human eggs *in vitro*, and published photographs of two- and four-cell human embryos in the American *Journal of Obstetrics and Gynecology*. They noted that the timing of the one-cell, two-cell and four-cell stages varied in time like those of other mammals. In 1955, Shettles[10] recognized that treatment of infertility was possible by IVF, an opinion shared by Rock, who commented that Shettles might be able to extract an egg from the ovary via a laparoscope, fertilize it *in vitro* and return it to the uterus: 'thus he [Shettles] will impregnate the woman in spite of the fact that she has no tubes'.

In the 1950s, a significant observation was made independently by the Australian Austin[11], and by Chang[12] working in the USA. Both workers demonstrated the requirement for spermatozoa to undergo certain changes, which endowed them with the capacity to fertilize. This process of 'capacitation' was a necessary step in the preparation of spermatozoa before fertilization could occur *in vitro*. However, in humans this was later observed to be unnecessary.

In 1954, penetration of the rabbit zona pellucida by spermatozoa, and pronuclear formation *in vitro*, were recorded by the microcinematographic study of McCarthy. By 1959 Chang had unequivocally demonstrated successful IVF in the rabbit.

More recent developments

In the early 1950s the first attempts were made at cooling embryos. In 1955 Chang and Morden investigated the effect of cooling preimplantation embryos to low temperatures. Smith reported 'exposure to very low temperatures is not incompatible with further development of mammalian eggs'. Chang and McDonough[13], in Massachusetts, USA, collected two-cell embryos from white rabbits, placed them in serum, lowered the temperature to 10°C in a vacuum flask, and then transported them to Cambridge, UK, where they were transferred to black recipient rabbit foster mothers. Eventually white, California-type rabbits were born. In 1972 Whittingham and colleagues[14] and, working independently, Wilmut[15], published their results on the cryopreservation, thawing and survival of mouse embryos. This work was to lead the way to the successful cryopreservation of human embryos.

Chang made further major contributions to the IVF process. By 1969 convincing evidence for successful IVF in mammals, with all criteria satisfied, had been established for the hamster, mouse and rabbit. During this period hormonal treatments were developed, leading to oocyte maturation and ovulation. In 1961, Katz and Herman[16–18] published their studies on hormonal treatments leading to the resumption of meiosis and ovulation in humans. In 1969, Edwards and co-workers[17] published a significant report on the sequence of events during human oocyte maturation, demonstrating the early stages of fertilization of the human oocyte. In 1970, Steptoe and associates[18] published a report on the first human blastocyst observed *in vitro*.

The work of Steptoe and Edwards led, in 1978, to the birth of the first human after conception *in vitro*[19]. The key developments in IVF are summarized in Table 1.1. Since that birth, an enormous amount of research has been carried out into the processes and procedures of IVF. However, it is a curious but significant anomaly that relatively few follow-up studies of the children produced by these techniques have been undertaken. Those involved in treating infertile couples often work in units without any allied input from pediatricians. Payment for treatment does not include payment for continuing assessment. Attitudes vary among fertility specialists concerning the issue of the health of IVF children, with many taking a constructive view to supporting the assessment of outcome. The following anecdote gives another position within the spectrum of 'responsibility–irresponsibility' encountered when considering follow-up or continuing assessment of children conceived after assisted reproductive technologies (ART). A famous medical institution in the USA, which I visited in late 2000, had a well-known (amongst pediatricians) relationship between those involved in the treatment of fertility and those involved in the treatment of premature babies. The leading neonatologist, out of exasperation, had promised a silver dollar (in the style of Moby Dick, who posted a silver dollar to the mast of his ship) to challenge *anyone* from the fertility unit to visit the neonatal intensive care unit. Nobody claimed the money.

Without wishing to parody the relationship between these colleagues, and being very much aware that there is nothing more indignant than a vested interest manifesting as a moral principle, it is clear from personal observations that such regrettable relationships do exist.

It is for these colleagues, for non-clinical scientists, for parents of children conceived with the help of ART, and for the purposes of refuting

Table 1.1 Key events in the development of *in vitro* fertilization (IVF)

Year	*Event*	*Key investigators involved*
1878	First attempts at *in vitro* fertilization in mammalian eggs	Schenk[1]
1891	First successful egg recovery from rabbit	Heap[2]
1880	First successful embryo culture	Onanoff[3]
1930	First successful IVF of mammalian eggs resulting in a live birth	Pincus[4]
1952	Time of ovulation established in humans using laparoscopy	Rock[7]
1935	First successfully fertilized human eggs *in vitro*	Menkin and Rock[9]
1970	First human blastocyst observed *in vitro*	Edwards and colleagues[18]
1972	Mouse embryo successfully cryopreserved and thawed, with survival	Wilmut[15]
1978	Birth of Louise Brown, first human born after IVF	Steptoe and Edwards[19]
1983	First pregnancy after replacement of cyropreserved embryo	Trounson[58]
1990	Preimplantation genetic diagnosis* first described	Handyside and colleagues[59]
1992	Intracytoplasmic sperm injection developed in humans	Palermo and colleagues[21]

* Although preimplantation genetic diagnosis is not a treatment *per se*, it does have ramifications for children and is therefore considered in this table

any myths created about these children (positive or negative) that this book has been written.

In vitro fertilization

It is not within the remit of this book to describe the IVF process in detail. However, some points that are worthy of note will be described here. IVF involves the harvesting of oocytes from the mother to be, using a laparoscope or, more latterly, ultrasound-guided transvaginal oocyte pickup using a needle. This is after treatment with powerful supraphysiological doses of gonadotropic hormones to 'guarantee' ovulation induction. A more detailed description is in Chapter 2. More recently, natural cycle IVF has been suggested in which the drugs are not used, in an effort to avoid exposure of the mother to known short-term complications (such as ovarian hyperstimulation syndrome) and the unknown long-term side-effects of these hormones. In reality, however, natural cycle IVF would make IVF less practical (for example timing egg recovery).

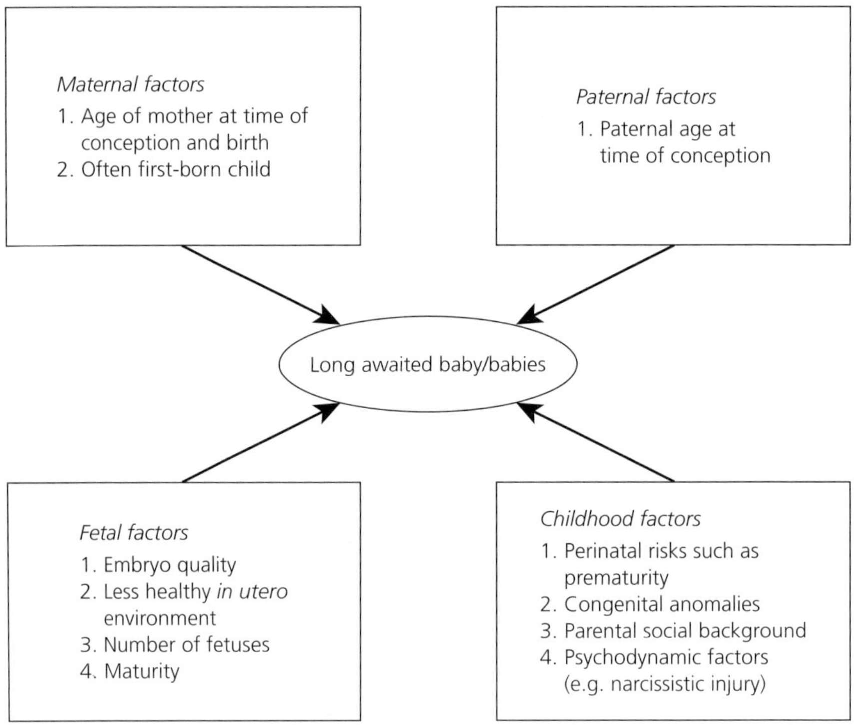

Figure 1.1 Some of the potential factors that may have a bearing on the well-being of *in vitro* fertilization children

The fresh ejaculated sperm, or in some cases freeze–thawed sperm, is then 'mixed' with the oocytes after sperm preparation. If normal fertilization occurs, up to three of the resulting embryos are transferred to the uterus 48 h after egg collection. This is a standard procedure in which a fine flexible catheter containing the embryos is passed through the cervix into the uterine cavity, and the embryos are expelled in a minimal quantity of medium.

The techniques involved in IVF have become more refined since its original invention, and novel forms of IVF have been developed. Prior to discussion of these it is worthwhile considering the theoretical risks to which all children conceived after IVF are exposed (Figure 1.1). Inevitably, factors that may be risks for children conceived from standard IVF conceptions will also generally be added on top of any distinct and separate factors related to the newer techniques discussed below.

Table 1.2 Theoretical risks to conceptions from embryo cryopreservation

Exposure to biochemical contaminants from the medium
Ice crystal formation within the embryo
Biochemical disturbance of the embryo structure, from propanediol, dimethylsulfoxide* or other chemicals used
Damage during thawing processes
Physical damage occurring during embryo manipulation for cryopreservation
Damage to DNA during embryo storage (the 'Winston' concept)

All the risks described in this table are more likely to lead to death of the embryo or developmental arrest rather than viable pregnancy
*Dimethylsulfoxide is now rarely used

NOVEL TECHNIQUES

Freezing

Although IVF with fresh embryo transfer has resulted in successful treatment for a large number of previously infertile couples, it is expensive and fails to be effective in cases of primary male infertility. In addition, embryo transfer was initially performed immediately after fertilization. However, if the procedure was successful and more than three embryos were created, these additional embryos would often be destroyed (transfer of three or more embryos conveys a significant risk of high-order multiple pregnancy). It is for these reasons, predominantly, that there was a need to develop other techniques, such as embryo cryopreservation and subsequent thawing. This technique is invaluable if the mother is thought to be developing ovarian hyperstimulation syndrome following embryo replacement. This condition is known to be exacerbated by pregnancy (and can be fatal). The severity of this complication of supraphysiological gonadotropin-induced ovulation can be reduced by deferring embryo transfer until a later cycle. Embryo cryopreservation also allows clinics to 'quarantine' embryos whilst screening egg or sperm donors for infectious diseases. The theoretical risks that arise from embryo cryopreservation are listed in Table 1.2.

Subzonal injection

The technique of partial zona dissection (PZD) was developed to increase the probability that a sperm capable of fertilization comes in contact with the oocyte. Although this method improved conventional IVF results, the improvement was only marginal and relatively large numbers of sperm are still required[20]. This drawback applied less to the subsequent technique of subzonal microinjection of spermatozoa (SUZI) into the perivitelline space. There is only one paper that has described pediatric outcome after SUZI and this is referred to in Chapter 4.

There is no literature specifically describing children conceived after PZD, which was a technique largely superceded by intracytoplasmic sperm injection (ICSI) and it is thus not further discussed. PZD, however, does share in common with preimplantation genetic diagnosis (PGD) and assisted hatching a risk factor related to the implicit manipulation of the zona pellucida in these techniques. It has been noted by some authors that any manipulation of the zona pellucida can result in an increased risk of monozygotic twinning in subsequent pregnancies. This is a major risk factor of these mainly new techniques, which will be discussed later.

Intracytoplasmic sperm injection

ICSI was first described by Palermo and colleagues in Belgium[21]. Its power as a technique has been such that its introduction has been very rapid. In ICSI a single spermatozoon is injected directly into the cytoplasm of the (harvested) egg using a fine glass needle. The sperm can be ejaculated, aspirated from the epididymis (trans-epididymal sperm aspiration, TESA) or collected directly from the testis (the latter two techniques requiring general anesthesia).

ICSI is used (in conjunction with conventional IVF) to overcome a variety of types of severe male-factor infertility or where infertility remains unexplained (often where conventional IVF alone has failed). The affected men suffer from low sperm counts, poor-quality sperm and/or poor sperm motility. Typically they have semen too poor for conventional IVF. In 2000 in the UK alone, there were already 78 centers licensed to use this method. Men benefiting from this treatment include those who have had a vasectomy reversed or chemotherapy, those with congenital abnormalities of the external genitalia (such as varicocele) and others with unexplained low sperm counts. In addition, ICSI is also useful in treating cases of infertility that have a genetic cause, such as translocations, Klinefelter's syndrome[22] and carriers of cystic fibrosis (CF) who often have absence of the vas deferens[23]. ICSI has also proved useful in men with testicular failure who may have small areas of testis with normal spermatogenesis. Such men can be treated by taking multiple fine-needle aspirate biopsies of the testis to identify normal areas, followed by the use of ICSI.

However, ICSI results in the bypassing of normal sperm selection techniques[24] and can also result in trauma to the sperm cytoskeleton.

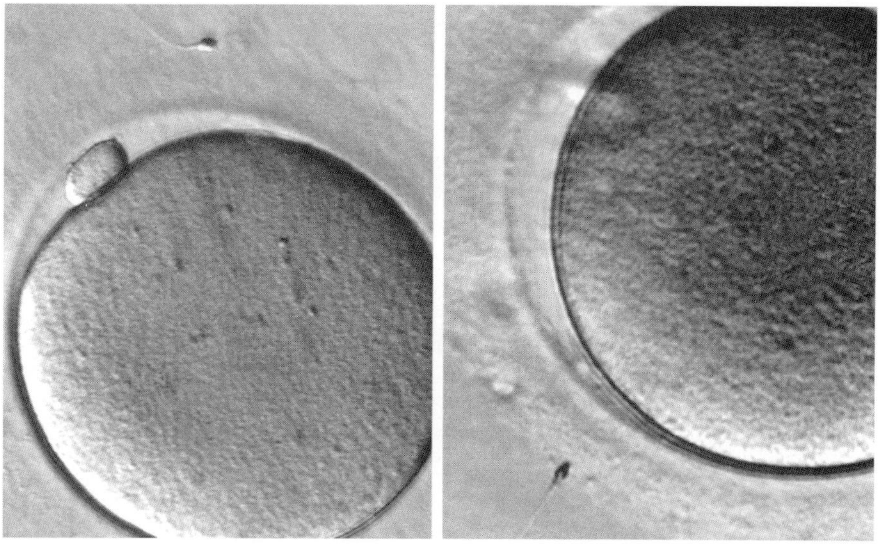

Figure 1.2 Mature oocytes and spermatozoa: the beginnings of a new life. Figure reproduced with kind permission of Dr Lucinda L. Veeck, MLT, hDSc, Cornell University Medical College, New York, USA

Chromosomal abnormalities have been noted in the sperm from men treated with ICSI[25]. Undoubtedly this adds to concern that this technological remedy for male infertility allows the injection of abnormal sperm, with untold consequences. In order to prevent the sperm tail from beating once it is inside the ovum, the selected sperm is immobilized just prior to injection by scraping over the sperm tail. Indeed it was this development by Fishel and associates[26] that paved the way for making ICSI successful. This scraping is thought to disturb the membrane potential of the sperm, immobilizing it, and the procedure appears to be beneficial for fertilization. The viscous agent that is used to slow the sperm down may cause chemical damage to the sperm. Whereas in normal conception the sperm does not enter the egg (Figure 1.2), in ICSI the entire sperm is injected into an egg denuded of cumulus cells. This involves piercing the outer and inner membranes of the egg and introducing a needle into it. The latest development, microinjection of round spermatid nuclei into oocytes (ROSNI) does not even require the completion of spermatogenesis[27]. The first birth after injection of testicle-derived spermatids was in 1995[28], but after this the technique was banned in the UK. For humans, the long-term consequences of bypassing the human spermatozoon's cytoplasmic contribution cannot yet be known[24].

Concerns about ICSI[24,29,30] can be categorized into five areas:

(1) The risks of using sperm that potentially carry genetic abnormalities;
(2) The risks of using sperm with structural defects;
(3) The potential for chemical and mechanical damage;
(4) The risk of introducing foreign material into the oocyte;
(5) The risk of bypassing sperm natural selection by the use of a single spermatozoon.

CONSIDERATION OF ALL THESE THERAPIES ACCORDING TO OUTCOME

From the pediatric perspective the outcome of ART, i.e. the birth of one or more children, can be considered in four categories:

(1) Congenital anomalies;
(2) Perinatal health/morbidity;
(3) Growth and neurodevelopmental well-being;
(4) Family relationships (in families where the parents have undergone often sustained infertility).

This book reviews the studies of children conceived after these various types of IVF and discusses these findings in the context of the above four categories. First, however, some considerations need to be discussed in more general terms when studies of IVF children are interpreted.

Congenital anomalies

Approximately 5% of all babies born in England and Wales are born with a congenital malformation or other developmental defect[31]. Many of these are noted at birth, but others only become apparent later. However, the UK national system of notification of infants with congenital malformations is restricted to conditions seen at birth or found in the first week of life[31]. Some malformations are incompatible with life, some can be corrected with surgery and others are compatible with continued life but cannot be corrected with treatment[32].

Congenital anomalies broadly arise via three mechanisms:

(1) Mutagenic, with the fetus inheriting a gene defect or chromosomal anomaly through their affected family or through a new mutation;
(2) At conception, including most non-inherited chromosomal anomalies;

(3) After conception, including teratogenic agents with non-heritable effects. The effect of any teratogen will depend on when in the pregnancy it acted, the strength of the dose and the fetal genetic susceptibility to that teratogen.

Relatively little is known about the cause of most congenital anomalies. Estimates suggest that approximately 14% are due to single mutant genes and major chromosomal abnormalities, about 5% are due to environmental factors (such as drugs and infections), a further 20% are due to the combined effects of environmental and genetic factors, but the cause of the remaining 60% or more of malformations remains unknown. As the infant mortality from other causes declines, congenital defects are accounting for an increasing proportion of infant deaths/morbidity and the search for causal factors has become more urgent. In the USA, for example, such malformations account for over 21% of infant mortality[33].

As stated in the short descriptions of IVF types at the beginning of this chapter, children conceived by ART could possibly be at increased risk for congenital anomalies. In assessing both pregnancy losses and congenital anomalies, a major underlying concern is that the ART population is not necessarily comparable to the general population.

First, the underlying infertility that necessitated ART may be associated with factors that persist and increase the rate of pregnancy loss or anomalies in the children. Frequency and severity of past illnesses are not necessarily comparable in the ART population and the general population. Infections producing tubal occlusion could persist in a chronic state. Women undergoing ART are usually older (mean age about 33 years[34]) than women conceiving naturally (mean age about 27 or 28 years[35]), and paternal age is also increased. Advanced maternal age is associated with increased risk of pregnancy loss[36,37] and liveborn aneuploidy[38,39], whereas advanced paternal age is associated with fresh Mendelian mutations[39–41]. Women undergoing ART and women in the general population also differ with respect to potential confounding variables such as maternal toxin exposure and nutrition. The higher maternal age in women undergoing ART places these women at increased risk compared with women in the general population, but lower exposure to toxins such as alcohol and cigarettes place the same women at decreased risk. The aggregate effect of these contradictory trends is uncertain.

Pregnancies conceived using ICSI from oligozoospermic men having Y deletions involving *DAZ* (deleted in azoospermia) genes illustrate that the

ART population differs from the general population in terms of likelihood of anomalies in liveborn children. Azoospermic men with Y deletions of the *DAZ* gene transmit the deleted Y to all male children, who will also be azoospermic or oligozoospermic. Thus, underlying genetic problems not only explain the infertility that caused a couple to seek ART, but place children at increased risk irrespective of the manner by which pregnancy was achieved – natural or ART.

Another example is that of men infertile because of congenital absence of the vas deferens (CAVD). Because a relationship exists between CAVD and mutations in the CF gene, a man with CAVD usually has two mutant CF alleles[41]. If the female is heterozygous for δF508, children could show δF508 CF homozygosity or compound heterozygosity (for more detailed discussion, see Chapter 4).

Pregnancy losses and conventional IVF

The frequency of spontaneous abortion was considered to be increased following IVF[42]. However, more recently following the observation that pregnancy in IVF is diagnosed earlier than in natural conception, figures from the Human Fertilisation and Embryology Authority (HFEA)[43] of the UK have suggested that abortion rates are similar to those of the normal population. Although it is assumed to be the result of hormonal imbalances adversely affecting implantation, an increased abortion rate is a potential concern, given that 50–60% of clinically recognized spontaneous abortions showed chromosomal abnormalities[44]. Cytogenetic abnormalities in ART have not been excluded as an explanation for the increased abortion rate. If chromosomal abnormalities contribute to the increased abortion rate, a corollary is that an increased risk would also exist for ART liveborns being cytogenetically abnormal.

Cohen and colleagues[45] collected details from 55 centers worldwide with 2329 IVF pregnancies; 577 (24.8%) resulted in early abortion, 36 in late abortion, three in therapeutic abortion and 120 in ectopic pregnancy. In the UK, the 430 IVF pregnancies reported from the Bourne–Hallam Medical Centre[46] included 93 cases (23%) that resulted in spontaneous abortion. In the USA cohort reported by the American Society of Reproductive Medicine (ASRM) and Society for Assisted Reproductive Technology[47] the spontaneous abortion rate was 18.6% in standard IVF, 18.9% and 21.6% with cryopreserved embryos. Data from the French National IVF Registry[48] showed consistent abortion rates of 16–20%. Data from the HFEA[43] showed a rate of 14%.

The 15–20% rate of spontaneous abortion in ART is generally considered to be elevated, but in fact this rate is barely increased over the background 'normal' rate of 14%[49].

Anomalies associated with conventional IVF

The opinion that congenital anomalies could be increased in ART pregnancies is plausible for several reasons, including:

(1) Selective mechanisms operating *in vivo* against morphologically abnormal sperm might not be comparably operative *in vitro*;
(2) An altered hormonal milieu *in vitro* may predispose to damage during meiosis or mitosis and hence cause chromosomal aneuploidy;
(3) Point mutations could result from the various chemical exposures inherent in extracorporeal fertilization.

Although surveys and registries have been set up to record these possible anomalies, a recurrent problem is that comparisons are being made to outcomes recorded in registries of birth defects, which are not necessarily the best comparison group. Although so far results have been reassuring (see Table 2.1), the problem is that disparate rates between centers suggest a lack of consistent criteria and data recording.

Spuriously increased rates

Examination following ART is often more rigorous than that following conventional pregnancy (controls). Unfortunately, this well-meaning medical surveillance can be scientifically misleading. Some anomalies such as small umbilical hernias, pigmented skin lesions and accessory auricles would not necessarily have been recorded in a registry of birth defects. It therefore follows that the ART anomaly rates might be spuriously overestimated. Although there are several internationally respected registries of birth defects, other less regimented collections of data can lead to underassessment of actual rates. Examples of the more vigorous surveillance for ART pregnancies include the UK Medical Research Council surveillance[50]. This records many anomalies not usually detected in neonatal surveys, such as mild hypospadias and undescended testes. A better comparison such as a prospective control study might involve analysis that takes into account the differing standards of record keeping.

Another assessment bias for ART children reflects the more detailed ultrasound scan usually performed in these pregnancies. For example, in the 1990 American Fertility Society/Society for Assisted Reproductive Technology (AFS/SART) cohort[51], probable abnormalities such as periventricular cyst, hydronephrosis, unilateral kidney agenesis, pyloric stenosis and pulmonary hypoplasia were noted. Such anomalies may not present until well after the first week of life, if ever. Finally, a subtler source of bias is the fact that continuing assessments are usually performed on the ART children after the early neonatal period. These can further contribute to the ascertained incompatibility with normal birth registries, by continuing to add anomalies to a list that is effectively closed in a standard registry.

Spuriously decreased rates

Failure to look systematically for congenital abnormalities Bias may also lead to lower than expected ART anomaly rates. In particular, an increased anomaly rate would not be recognized if ART centers did not systematically assess children for congenital anomalies. As an example, review of hospital case notes would be a poor way of ascertaining anomalies. Casual surveillance could explain the low anomaly rate recorded in certain surveys, for example 0.7% in Greek cases recorded by Cohen and associates[45], or 0.9% in the 1990 AFS/SART cohort[51]. The failure to search systematically for anomalies is a valid concern in almost all ART cohorts, with the notable exception of the small IVF case–control study of Morin and co-workers[52] and the ICSI cohort in Brussels[53].

Completeness of follow-up Another pitfall arises whenever a significant proportion of a given sample is lost to follow-up. One cannot assume that cases lost to follow-up are comparable with cases remaining for analysis. Moreover, the direction of bias is uncertain. Women lost to follow-up might not wish to be troubled because their children were healthy and because no personal benefit seemed to accrue from participating in a research protocol. The net effect would be a spuriously increased anomaly rate following ART because of the exclusion of normal outcomes. Conversely, women lost to follow-up who have experienced a bad outcome (pregnancy loss or birth of an anomalous infant) may resent the invasion of privacy or in some way blame an ART center and therefore fail to respond to requests for follow-up. Thus, the anomaly rate would be spuriously decreased.

If only a small proportion of cases from a large cohort are lost to follow-up, the remaining subjects could be assumed to be representative. However, this assumption is not necessarily valid when the outcome sought is infrequent or when a relatively high proportion of cases is lost to follow-up.

In ART surveillance the number of cases lost to follow-up may be several-fold greater than the background 4–5% anomaly rate. In the 1998 AFS/SART report[54], 58 anomalies were reported in 3873 babies (1.5%), yet 447 of the babies were lost to follow-up (11.5%). If even 10% of the 447 lost cases were anomalous, overall anomaly rates would have risen to 2.7%. In the most recent HFEA report[43] it was claimed that only 0.8% of all children born from IVF were born with an abnormality. However, this figure was obtained by relying on centers recording and reporting this information. Often children are born away from their fertility treatment center, thus making the likelihood of such records being valid even more remote.

Inclusions and exclusions A common methodological shortcoming in ART surveillance is the pooling of anomalies in neonates with anomalies in abortuses (spontaneous or induced). These may include those abnormalities detected because of increased pregnancy surveillance, but not those abnormal fetuses discreetly aborted in private clinics. Birth defect registries do not record anomalies in abortuses, induced or spontaneous. The rate of chromosomal abnormalities in newborn infants, which is about 0.6%, is one-tenth of that found in abortuses of 5–12 weeks' gestational age[55]. Failure to document anomalies in induced abortuses is based not only on concerns about incomplete ascertainment, but also on knowledge that fetuses with anomalies may or may not have survived until birth. The natural history of anomalies is uncertain. For example, considerably fewer than half the trisomy 18 cases detected at amniocentesis survive until birth, and only two-thirds of trisomy 21 cases survive[55]. Pooling anomalies identified during prenatal cytogenetic surveillance (chorionic villus sampling, amniocentesis) with those detected at birth would thus yield data not comparable to the liveborn general population, although they would provide more complete outcome data for procedures such as ART, albeit with uncertain and probably incomplete information regarding 'normal' pregnancies.

Perinatal health or morbidity

There are a variety of factors, which pertain to ART pregnancies of all types, that increase risks to the newborn child, including the possibly higher rates of congenital anomalies discussed above. The supraphysiological gonadotropin regimes resulting in multiple egg release followed by the availability post-fertilization of multiple embryos result in the obvious temptation to replace more than one embryo. This will often be with the complicity of both the IVF clinical team and the expectant parents.

However, despite counselling, if one tells a couple that they may conceive triplets when they have not conceived at all for 10 years *they may not believe the counsellor*.

The known impact on multiple birth rates of IVF is discussed in more detail later (in Chapter 2). The implications of this higher frequency of multiple births for the child are profound, and increase with increasing sib numbers. These risks mainly manifest as the risks of prematurity and low birth weight.

However, there are now some positive developments that may result in a reduced risk of higher-order births. The use of natural-cycle IVF, the use of embryo scoring to replace only 'viable' embryos and the development of extended embryo culture will all result in reduced morbidity and mortality for IVF children. Some nations such as Australia and New Zealand have regulated a maximum two-embryo replacement. In the UK the evidence is consistent from the HFEA reports that the only effect of replacing three embryos is a higher rate of triplets, but paradoxically not an overall higher pregnancy rate. In so-called fetal reduction or selective abortion, where a multiple pregnancy is reduced to twins or a singleton, the very process itself will expose the surviving baby(ies) to risks not only of premature labor but also of embolization at the moment of abortion. The frequency of higher-order multiples (three, four or more) between 1973 and 1990 increased at approximately seven times that of singleton births. Whereas triplets and higher-order multiple births represented only 1.6% of all births in 1973, they accounted for 3.1% of all multiple births in 1990[56] in the USA.

Growth and neurodevelopmental well-being

One of the problems with considering the growth and neurodevelopmental well-being of IVF children is the difficulty of performing such studies. Whilst there is a small but dedicated group of individuals (of which I consider myself to be one!) who have performed studies on these children to varying ages and of varying detail, they have all come up against similar hurdles. These are best exemplified by a comment made at a recent presentation concerning the outcome of the latest national trial of chemotherapy for childhood acute lymphoblastic leukemia (UK ALL XI). Treatment of this condition has progressed enormously as a consequence of this national trial, into which every child who develops ALL is entered. However, among the long-term risks of treatment are secondary malignancies and neurodevelopmental difficulties. These children are systematically followed-up. However, the speaker at the presentation noted the difficulty involved in getting families to attend even a 5-yearly follow-up. One would think that, of all the groups who would be likely to come back again and again, this would be the group.

In IVF outcome studies the clinic that requests the review is often welcomed by families ('Why didn't they contact us sooner?') and in my experience also often benefits from a 'halo effect' ('They gave us our child'). But the validity of such studies is weakened immensely by the absence of a control group, and it is recruiting a control group that is often difficult. While many families with children from ART are by their very nature 'winners' in an exacting and psychologically stressful process, other families need to be persuaded to help. Systematic follow-up of children conceived after these various forms of ART is performed by few centers and even those suffer from non-attendance.

Neurodevelopmentally these children experience both positive and negative influences on their well-being. On the 'downside' they are often born earlier with a lower mean birth weight, sometimes from multiple births, to older mothers. On the 'upside' they are often born to families with greater means and of higher socioeconomic status (these factors allow families to pay for their treatment in the first place.) A full discussion of these factors and their scientific validity is presented in Chapter 2.

Growth is a simpler issue. There are national growth parameters. Providing that valid account is taken of parental heights, and that measurements are both standardized and serial, any long-term growth effects on the ART-conceived child can easily be ascertained. The expression 'growth is a bioassay of well-being' is most important in considering the significance of growth and its normality as a measure of the effect of any intervention which may affect the health of a child.

Family relationships

An often quoted myth is that IVF children are more *wanted* than naturally conceived children. This idea arose from a paper written in a very early study of IVF children[57] that is still repeated despite, in my opinion, being based on weak science. In a way the repetition of this myth is symptomatic of much literature published about ART-conceived children. Like it or not, studies on these children often attract widespread publicity, especially if their findings are in any way unusual. My aim in writing this book is to concentrate on reviewed and qualified worldwide studies concerning children conceived after ART for the benefit of all involved in their care.

REFERENCES

1. Schenk SL. Das saugethieri kuntslich befruchtet ausserhalb desmutterthieres. *Mitt Embryol Inst Wein* 1878;1:107
2. Heap W. Preliminary note on the transplantation and growth of mammalian ova within a uterine foster mother. *Proc R Soc* 1891;48:457–8
3. Onanoff M. *CR Soc Biol* 1880:719
4. Pincus G. The comparative behaviour of mammalian eggs *in vivo* and *in vitro* – the development of fertilised and artificially activated rabbit eggs. *Proc R Soc* 1930;85–132
5. Pincus G, Enzmann E. Comparative behavior of mammalian eggs *in vivo* and *in vitro*; activation of ovarian eggs. *J Exp Med* 1935;62:665
6. Pincus G, Saunders B. The comparative behaviour of mammalian eggs *in vivo* and *in vitro*. *Anat Rec* 1939;75:537–45
7. Rock (1952) cited in Fishel S, Symonds EM, eds. *IVF – Past Present Future*. Oxford: IRL Press, 1986
8. Lewis G (1956) cited in Fishel S, Symonds EM, eds. *IVF – Past Present Future*. Oxford: IRL Press, 1986
9. Menkin M, Rock J. *In vitro* fertilisation and cleavage of human ovarian eggs. *J Obstet Gynaecol* 1935;55:440–52
10. Shettles L. Further observations on living human oocytes and ova. *Am J Obstet Gynecol* 1955;69:365–71
11. Austin C. Observation on the penetration of the sperm into the mammalian egg. *Aust J Sci Res* 1951;B4:581
12. Chang M. Fertilization of rabbit ova *in vitro*. *Nature (London)* 1959;184:406
13. Chang M, McDonough J. An experiment to cross the cottontail and the domestic rabbit. *J Hered* 1955;56:41–4
14. Whittingham DG, Lyon MF, Glenister PH. Long-term storage of mouse embryos at –196 degrees C: the effect of background radiation. *Genet Res* 1977;29:171–81
15. Wilmut I. Effect of cooling rate, warming rate, cryoprotective agent and stage of development on survival of mouse embryos during the freezing and thawing. *Life Sci* 1972;11:1071–9
16. Katz, Herman (1961) cited in Fishel S, Symonds EM, eds. *IVF – Past Present Future*. Oxford: IRL Press, 1986
17. Edwards R, Bavister G, Steptoe P. Early stages of fertilization *in vitro* of human oocytes matured *in vitro*. *Nature (London)* 1969;221:632
18. Edwards R, Steptoe P, Purdy J. Fertilization and cleavage *in vitro* of preovulatory human oocytes. *Nature (London)* 1970;227:1307
19. Steptoe PC, Edwards RG. Birth after the reimplantation of a human embryo. *Lancet* 1978;2:366
20. van Rumste MM, Evers JL, Farquhar CM, Blake DA. Intra-cytoplasmic sperm injection versus partial zona dissection, subzonal insemination and conventional techniques for oocyte insemination during *in vitro* fertilisation. *Cochrane Database Syst Rev* 2000;(2):CD001301
21. Palermo G, Joris H, Devroey P, Van Steirteghem AC. Pregnancies after intracytoplasmic injection of single spermatozoon into an oocyte. *Lancet* 1992;340:17–18
22. Tournaye H, Staessen C, Liebaers I, *et al*. Testicular sperm recovery in nine 47,XXY Klinefelter patients. *Hum Reprod* 1996;11:1644–9
23. Schlegel PN, Cohen J, Goldstein M, *et al*. Cystic fibrosis gene mutations do not affect sperm function during *in vitro* fertilization with micromanipulation for men with bilateral congenital absence of vas deferens. *Fertil Steril* 1995;64:421–6

24. Cummins JM, Jequier AM. Concerns and recommendations for intracytoplasmic sperm injection (ICSI) treatment. *Hum Reprod* 1995;10(suppl 1):138–43
25. Jaffe T, Oates RD. Genetic abnormalities and reproductive failure. *Urol Clin North Am* 1994;21:389–408
26. Fishel S, Lisi F, Rinaldi L, *et al*. Systematic examination of immobilizing spermatozoa before intracytoplasmic sperm injection in the human. *Hum Reprod* 1995;10:497–500
27. Sofikitis N, Miyagawa I, Yamamoto Y, Loutradis D, Mantzavinos T, Tarlatzis V. Micro- and macro-consequences of ooplasmic injections of early haploid male gametes. *Hum Reprod Update* 1998;4:197–212
28. Fishel S, Green S, Bishop M, *et al*. Pregnancy after intracytoplasmic injection of spermatid. *Lancet* 1995;345:1641–2
29. Patrizio P. Intracytoplasmic sperm injection (ICSI): potential genetic concerns. *Hum Reprod* 1995;10:2520–3
30. De Kretser DM. The potential of intracytoplasmic sperm injection (ICSI) to transmit genetic defects causing male infertility. *Reprod Fertil Dev* 1995;7:137–42
31. Templeton A, Morris JK. Reducing the risk of multiple births by transfer of two embryos after *in vitro* fertilization. *New Engl J Med* 1998;339:573–7
32. Botting B. Congenital anomalies. In *The Health of our Children*. London: HMSO, 1997:148–58
33. Windham GC, Edmonds LD. Current trends in the incidence of neural tube defects. *Pediatrics* 1982;70:333–7
34. Angell RR. Aneuploidy in older women: higher rates of aneuploidy in oocytes from older women. *Hum Reprod* 1994;9:1199–201
35. Office of Population Censuses and Surveys 1998. London: HMSO, 1998
36. Smith KE, Buyalos RB. The profound impact of patient age on pregnancy outcome after early detection of fetal cardiac activity. *Fertil Steril* 1996;65:35–40
37. Hassold T, Abruzzo M, Adkins K, *et al*. Human aneuploidy: incidence, origin and aetiology. *Environ Mol Mutagen* 1996;28:167–75
38. Wyrobek AJ, Aardema M, Eichenlaub-Ritter U, *et al*. Mechanisms and targets involved in maternal and paternal age effects on numerical aneuploidy. *Environ Mol Mutagen* 1996;28:254–64
39. McIntosh GC, Olshan A, Baird PA. Paternal age and the risk of birth defects in offspring. *Epidemiology* 1995;6:282–8
40. Yoshida A, Miura K, Shirai M. Cytogenetic survey of 1007 infertile males. *Urol Int* 1997;58:166–76
41. Patrizio P, Asch RH, Handelin B, Silber SJ. Aetiology of congenital absence of vas deferens; genetic study of three generations. *Hum Reprod* 1993;8:215–20
42. Saunders DM, Lancaster P. The wider perinatal significance of the Australian *in vitro* fertilization data collection program. *Am J Perinatol* 1989;6:252–5
43. Seventh Annual Human Fertilisation and Embryology Authority Report. London: HFEA, 1998
44. Boue A, Boue J. Chromosome abnormalities and abortion. *Basic Life Sci* 1974;4: 317–39
45. Cohen J, Mayaux MJ, Guihard-Moscato ML. Pregnancy outcomes after *in vitro* fertilization. A collaborative study on 2342 pregnancies. *Ann NY Acad Sci* 1988;541:1–6
46. Rizk B, Doyle P, Tan SL, *et al*. Perinatal outcome and congenital malformations in *in-vitro* fertilization babies from the Bourn–Hallam group. *Hum Reprod* 1991;6: 1259–64
47. Steinberg EP, Holtz PM, Sullivan EM, Villar CP. Profiling assisted reproductive technology: outcomes and quality of infertility management. *Fertil Steril* 1998;69: 617–23

48. French National IVF Registry: analysis of 1986 to 1990 data. FIVNAT (French *In Vitro* National). *Fertil Steril*. 1993;59:587–95
49. Simpson JL, Liebaers I. Assessing congenital anomalies after preimplantation genetic diagnosis. *J Assist Reprod Genet* 1996;13:170–6
50. Doyle P, Beral V, Maconochie N. Preterm delivery, low birthweight and small-for gestational age in liveborn singleton babies resulting from *in-vitro* fertilization. *Hum Reprod* 1992;7:425–8
51. Medical Research International, Society for Assisted Reproductive Technology (SART), The American Fertility Society. *In vitro* fertilization–embryo transfer (IVF-ET) in the United States: 1990 results from the IVF–ET Registry. *Fertil Steril* 1992;57:15–24
52. Morin NC, Wirth H, Johnson DH, *et al*. Congenital malformations and psychosocial development in children conceived by *in vitro* fertilisation. *J Pediatr* 1989;115: 222–7
53. Bonduelle M, Joris H, Hofmans K, Liebaers I, van Steirteghem A. Mental development of 201 ICSI children at 2 years of age. *Lancet* 1998;351:1553
54. Assisted reproductive technology in the United States and Canada: 1995 results generated from the American Society for Reproductive Medicine/Society for Assisted Reproductive Technology Registry. *Fertil Steril* 1998;69:389–98
55. Yamamoto M, Watanabe G. Epidemiology of gross chromosomal anomalies at the early embryonic stage of pregnancy. *Cont Epidemiol Biostat* 1979;1:101–6
56. Luke B. The changing pattern of multiple births in the United States: maternal and infant characteristics, 1973 and 1990. *Obstet Gynecol* 1994;84:101–6
57. Golombok S. Psychological functioning in infertility patients. *Hum Reprod* 1992; 7:208–12
58. Trounson A. Human pregnancy following cryopreservation, thawing and transfer of an eight-cell embryo. *Nature (London)* 1983;305:707–9
59. Handyside AH, Kontogianni EH, Hardy K, Winston RM. Pregnancies from biopsied human preimplantation embryos sexed by Y-specific DNA amplification. *Nature (London)* 1990;344:768–70

2

A review of studies investigating outcome in IVF children

'I am I plus my circumstances'

José Ortega y Gasset,[1] 1955

The first IVF child (Louise Brown) is now 23 years old, so the knowledge of the ultimate outcome (the growth of IVF children into healthy adults) is immediately limited to the knowledge of, at best, young adults. The largest group of IVF-conceived individuals are still in childhood; they are the 'first generation'. This review attempts to guide the reader to an overview of known outcomes whilst attributing scientific limitations to those studies. Before this, however, a brief description of IVF seems apt[1].

Most IVF starts with programmed superovulation schedules. This allows oocyte retrieval to occur on specific days of the week in 'batches'. A standard protocol (of which there are many variations) uses down-regulation with gonadotropin releasing hormone agonist, commencing in the luteal phase of the previous cycle, and ovarian stimulation with purified follicle stimulating hormone (FSH) by subcutaneous injection. Ovulation is then induced by subcutaneous administration of human chorionic gonadotropin (hCG). Oocyte retrieval performed by vacuum aspiration of follicles under vaginal ultrasound guidance is usually scheduled for 34–36 h later. Oocytes are routinely inseminated with a concentration of normal motile sperm of 100 000/ml. However, this will be increased with sperm with suboptimal characteristics (see also Chapter 4). Fertilization is then scored at 17–20 h and embryo transfer is carried out at 48–54 h, although more recently earlier transfer has become possible. Indeed, after intracytoplasmic sperm injection (ICSI), activated oocytes can be transferred within 1 h to the uterus. It can be seen from this brief description that this process is quite different from natural conception!

WHAT IS KNOWN ABOUT IVF CHILDREN – SOME QUALIFYING COMMENTS

To inform the following review the reader may wish to consider common errors in research methodology that limit the validity of some of the findings of any outcome studies performed on IVF children.

These are best divided into errors that are seen in neurodevelopmental outcome studies and those looking more at congenital anomalies.

Errors in neurodevelopmental outcome studies

(1) *Unstandardized tools:* if a child is assessed using a system for which norms have not been established for that population (e.g. American system used in Australia) then results could be misleading;
(2) *Multiple observers:* interobserver error is a common problem;
(3) *Poor matching criteria:* control groups need to be matched for factors that may have a profound effect on the child's performance, e.g. socioeconomic status, separate from the outcome being studied;
(4) *Poor follow-up rates:* a rate of 80% or above is more likely to be representative. If a follow-up rate is poor, any factor that may differ with the assessed children needs to be established;
(5) *Insufficient power:* with standardized tools of assessment (e.g. Griffiths scales of mental development; Figure 2.1) it is possible to predict the numbers of children needed for a certain strength/reliability for that conclusion;
(6) *Absence of a control group:* with smaller studies, controls are critical;
(7) *Inappropriate control group:* it is assumed that the IVF couple would like to know how their child compares with naturally conceived children, not with other types of IVF children (e.g. comparing ICSI with IVF);
(8) *Insensitive tools of assessment:* assessing development by telephone questionnaires is unlikely to reveal much.

Errors in congenital anomaly studies

(1) *Including data from abortions:* this is potentially useful, but only if the comparison group has a similar level of data ascertainment (in reality unlikely);

(2) *Including data from children over the age of 1 week:* as stated elsewhere, about 30% of anomalies are not detected until after 1 week of age, so if these are included this may have the effect of introducing a bias in the results;
(3) *Comparing 'apples with oranges':* if, for example, congenital anomaly figures from a cohort of children born in country *y* and incidence of anomalies are compared with those from country *z* this may introduce a bias, due to such things as different racial mix;
(4) *Over-ascertainment:* for example, the inclusion of ultrasound scans in the studied group but not in the comparison group.

Disturbingly, one often hears of 'report A' or 'report B' interpreted as meaning 'E' when in fact, because of their limitations, they really mean 'C'. The main problem is that pediatric outcome is both difficult to measure and expensive. Furthermore, it often relies on the goodwill and motivation of families who have benefited from fertility treatments. Most of these families have great pride in their children, which motivates them to share information with others. Other families, whilst still proud of their children, wish for various reasons to keep the nature of their child's conception to themselves. Even where there have been meaningful studies with larger numbers of children, attracting control groups for comparison is often difficult. Snowden and Snowden[1], in their research, raised another difficulty: that the non-response rate increased markedly as the children became older (these were children conceived after donor insemination).

This review is divided into several sections: those that study early childhood and development; those that investigate neonatal outcomes; and those that look at a broader picture of the child in the context of the family and family relations.

PSYCHOSOCIAL OUTCOMES

Van Balen noted in 1998[2] that IVF had been a discovery that had made a radical change in human existence. He stated that there are four assumptions to make about IVF and parenting:

(1) IVF infants are seen as very 'precious' and this leads to overprotection by the parents;
(2) Parents have exaggerated expectations of their child, because they have taken so many efforts to have him or her;

(3) After a long period of infertility, parents cannot adapt to the hard reality of child-rearing practices. This causes them to experience more problems in the process of child rearing;
(4) The IVF child is seen as unusual or different by other people in his or her parents' environment.

Fortunately, there is very little evidence to support these hypotheses.

Studies that have looked at the consequences for children have lagged far behind, in part due to the rapid pace of advances. Whilst the new technology is exciting and has a powerful clientele wishing to advance it, the outcome studies are less exciting and more labor intensive, and infringe on an individual's privacy. To address concerns that conception by IVF may have a negative effect on a child's cognitive and emotional development, or possibly the quality of parent–child relationships, there have been a group of researchers who have pursued this area of enquiry and their work is reviewed here. This review tends to concentrate on individuals who have specialized in this area. Referrals in more general terms to the literature that supports their area of investigation are avoided, partly because this is full of contradictions and partly because it is beyond the scope of this book.

FAMILY RELATIONSHIPS

In addition to concerns about child development, IVF and especially ICSI is likely to be associated with increased parental stress, compared to normal conception, which may adversely affect both child development and family relationships. McWhinnie[3] has suggested two areas of strain on parenthood pertinent to ICSI: first, the impact of male infertility and the subsequent deception of the child; and second, the dilemma of revealing or maintaining a secret for a lifetime from children, relatives or friends. Colpin and co-workers[4] argued that the unusual form of the transition to parenthood in cases of artificial reproduction could profoundly influence the attitudes and expectations of parents towards their child and consequently the nature of the ensuing parent–child attachment. Parents at particular risk may be those who have not worked through their conflict towards infertility, in which case the child may act as a 'narcissistic injury'[5], constantly reminding at least one parent of her or his infertility and possibly creating an asymmetry between the parents[4]. In addition, Colpin and colleagues emphasized that, apart from the medical context and the artificial character of the conception, pregnancy achieved by IVF can be extremely stressful, with a low conception rate and an increased risk of multiple pregnancy, spontaneous abortion and death after premature delivery. Having endured long periods of waiting and uncertainty about the survival of their child, parents may either hesitate to bond with their baby[6] or become insecurely attached, with the associated risks of overprotection[4] and disregard for the child's need to develop autonomy.

In view of this research, it seems pertinent to review the studies that have investigated family relations to date, and try to summarize their message. Golombok and colleagues[7], in a series of papers on 'families created by the new reproductive technologies', investigated 41 IVF families and 45 families conceived by donor insemination (DI) with controls of 43 naturally conceived children and 55 families with a child adopted at birth. This was a study very early in the progress of IVF, with only 200 children having reached the age range for the study (4–8 years). A variety of measures were applied to this small group of children. These aimed to look at parents' marital and psychological state, quality of parenting, and children's emotions, behavior and relationships. Critically the examiners in this study were not blinded to the mode of conception and no power calculation to measure strength of conclusions was recorded. The conclusion that IVF families' quality of parenting was better than that of families with a naturally conceived child was not surprising, in view of the design errors of the study. A larger group with a blinded examiner would be more likely to draw valid conclusions. Such a study is ongoing, involving groups in the UK, Belgium, Denmark, Sweden and Greece. This will assess family relations in 650 IVF, 650 ICSI and 650 naturally conceived children and will have a psychologist in each arm of the project blinded to the mode of conception. Because the views of Golombok's early study were particularly attractive to IVF families (that their children were more 'wanted' than naturally conceived children) and to the clinics treating these couples, the message of this rather weak study has been repeated often. Golombok extended her work to a European group, in which there were 111 participants from the UK, the Netherlands, Spain and Italy[7]. Again there were control groups that included adoptive families (115) and naturally conceived children (120). Again, blinding was not applied and the conclusions of the study supported those of her earlier British paper mentioned above[7]. It should be noted that the response rate amongst DI families in the British study was 62% and in the European study 47%.

There is a tendency for those in research to find what they intend to find, and the only way this bias, conscious or otherwise, can be overcome is by good study design. In some of my own work in this field blinding was not applied; however, there were other reasons for this and it could be argued that the majority of outcomes I was looking for could be assessed without relying on subtle judgements. In Golombok's work the forms/questionnaires used needed to be scored. It is this very scoring that could be biased, if someone knew from which group the child came.

Golombok has also looked at children raised in fatherless families[7]. Here she compared 30 lesbian mother families with 42 single mother families and 42 heterosexual families. Here she relied on lesbian volunteers for that group but not the heterosexual group, and in addition did not use blinding for maternal outcomes. The measures used were not standardized against lesbian couples as a group and it is therefore impossible to say what the 'norms' are in this group. The conclusions here were that children raised in fatherless families experienced greater warmth and interaction with their mother, and were more securely attached to her, but perceived themselves to be less cognitively and physically competent than their peers from father-present families. It is worthy of note that in the UK the Human Fertilisation and Embryology Act 1990 requires the welfare of the child to be considered, including the need of that child for a father, in the decision of whether or not to offer assisted reproduction, although there are no specific criteria for acceptance or rejection of prospective parents.

In a study by Cook and colleagues[8], parenting quality, parental stress and child behavior in families with twins conceived by IVF were compared with families with naturally conceived twins. Here only 12 families were compared with 14 naturally conceived children. In this preliminary study, higher levels of stress were found in IVF families. However, the majority of IVF twins were first born in this group and possibly the greater experience of parenting of the naturally conceived children's parents helped reduce their stress levels.

Finally, Golombok investigated social versus biological parenting[7] via families where socioemotional development of children conceived by egg or sperm donation was compared with adoptive families. In this study of 41 such families, differences were noted between parents according to their genetic relationship with their child. Where children were not genetically related to their mother, there was higher maternal satisfaction than when they were not genetically related to their father.

McWhinnie and team in Dundee spent many years delving into the subject of family relations and IVF children and produced some interesting reports. Whilst many of these are elegant discussions reflecting McWhinnie's previous interests in adopted children, she has performed a study[9] looking at outcome for families created by assisted conception programs. In this study she makes a very pertinent observation. Reactions to infertility were despair, isolation, anger, envy of others and a hidden grief. Almost all reported that, on learning of infertility, the infertile person told their partner that they should leave them and find an alternative mate. The reaction of men told that they could never father children ranged from devastation to blind rage.

This descriptive study of 43 children from IVF and gamete intrafollicular transfer (GIFT) from the families interviewed were all reported as developing within normal limits. However, families were concerned that their child may be singled out as unusual or bizarre and this has led to varying levels of secrecy about involvement with an IVF program at all. The term 'test-tube baby' is disliked by many as inaccurate and a label. Thirty-five per cent of the IVF families did not use it in any reference to their child. Also, the medical language of infertility and assisted conception regimes can be misconstrued and be experienced as at variance with the medical meaning of the terms. For example, the selection of the 'best eggs' or 'best embryos' can produce fantasy about the potential development of these children. One family who participated in my first study of children born after embryo cryopreservation highlighted to me the harsh reality of some families' views about IVF conception, that they want a perfect baby, not just a baby. This particular family had twins whom I met at the age of about 14 months. One of these little ones clearly had clinical rickets with bowing of the tibia and delayed walking. At this time the affected twin was diagnosed with a genetic cause of rickets, hypophosphatemic rickets. This is an eminently treatable condition, which merely involves giving special vitamin D preparations. The outcome for any child with this problem is a healthy life with normal life expectancy, no residual disability and no major treatment requirement. The family were wealthy and could not have any financial reason for wanting not to have such a child in the future. She was a beautiful little girl. But nonetheless I heard later that the outstanding frozen embryos that were in storage would be tested for this condition (on the family's request) before any were to be replaced. My eyes were opened!

Mushin and co-workers[5] suggested that, because of the long periods of waiting and investment in having the child, parents may develop unreasonably high expectations. The risk is that parents will expect their long-awaited child to compensate for all the suffering they have gone through, but this is a desire that no child can fulfil[10]. The parents may then be disappointed when forced to confront the practicalities of parenting. Some IVF clinics have addressed this issue and have produced supportive family-friendly literature, which acknowledges, 'being pregnant was so exciting and now the more demanding … mundane task of bringing up your little one is upon you'.

Colpin and associates[4] studied parent–child relationships and the parents' psychosocial functioning in families which had a first-born child and compared this child with a non-matched naturally conceived control child. This study was unusual in that it involved observations of the parent–child relationship in the family home. It had been suggested that the unusual form of the transition to parenthood in cases of artificial reproduction could influence both the attitudes and the expectations of parents towards their child and the nature of the parent–child attachment[11]. Reassuringly, in this later study the relationship between these mothers and their children did not seem to differ from the natural situation. This finding was in line with studies by Golombok and colleagues[7] and Raoul-Duval and colleagues[12]. Work is ongoing in this area of enquiry. The most recent report[13], which studied 3–7 year olds from Taiwan, although typically there were a modest number of cases (54 IVF mother–child pairs and 59 naturally conceived mother–child pairs), concluded that parents showed somewhat greater emotional involvement, including warmth and protectiveness, with children conceived through IVF, and these parents were not more hesitant to set limits.

PERINATAL OUTCOME FOR IVF INFANTS

It has long been recognized that IVF children are at greater risk of perinatal morbidity. These risks result from being born less mature and of lower birth weight. The major effect is from the higher rate of twins, triplets and more in these conceptions. Quality data are from large studies and these will mainly be concentrated on when the findings are interpreted. A number of birth registries have been established, some of which were set up as a record of that particular country's fertility treatment, whereas others are reports from national data in which IVF births have been selected from of data on all births. The advantage of the latter data is that they can be compared more easily with the whole population. The disadvantage is that ascertainment of factors that may later prove important (e.g. hormones used in ovulation induction) may not be possible. The more focused specialist registries may be weak for certain specific abnormalities. For example, if one were looking at a rare abnormality such as Beckwith–Weidemann syndrome, which occurs in approximately 1 in 14 500 births[14], then in a country with a small population such as Sweden or Israel it would take a long time for any difference in the

Table 2.1 A few summary statistics concerning large studies of IVF outcome at birth

Country	*Type of registry*	*Mean gestation at birth*	*Frequency of multiple births*	*Mean birth weight*
France[15]	all births 1987–89 from 11 centers	22.7% of all births and 12.2% of singletons preterm (France has 5.6% of singletons born prematurely)	45% of children! 1669 births of which 582 were twins and 171 were triplets or higher	3.095 kg singletons, 2.363 kg twins
Belgium[16]	Dutch-speaking Belgium, all births 1992–97	22.2% preterm but in normal population only 5.58% preterm	not recorded	3172 g singleton IVF vs. 3314 g singleton naturally conceived
France[17]	national registry, but only 80% of IVF-ET recorded 1986–90	29.3% preterm	26.8% multiple births	2.718 kg singletons
Denmark[18]	national IVF registry 1994–95	23.8% preterm but with matched control group allowing for twins, etc., 23.4% in this group	similar to control groups	2992 g in the IVF group, 2996 g in the control group (NS)
Sweden[19]	retrospective cohort study of all Swedish births	30.3% IVF preterm vs. 6.3% controls	27% multiple births (1% in the control groups)	not recorded
Israel[20]	national survey, 1982–89	28.6% preterm	23.6% multiple births	2.873 kg IVF, 3.221 kg control group
UK[21]	national survey, 1978–87	24% preterm	23% multiple births	mean birth weights not stated but were lower than naturally conceived

IVF–ET, *in vitro* fertilization and embryo transfer

IVF population to be noted in relation to the rest of the population. Specialist registries are sometimes prone to another type of error: in some countries participation in them by clinics is not compulsory (e.g. SART in the USA).

The findings of these birth registry reports are summarized in Table 2.1[15–21]. This was a difficult table to construct, because each paper had a different way of presenting data. It is clear, however, that the babies born after IVF were more likely to be born before their due date, and this is mainly a result of there being more multiple births. Even with singleton births, it has been shown that IVF babies are likely to be born earlier, although on average this may be only by a few days. These singleton IVF children are also likely to be a little lower in birth weight.

These facts are unlikely to be due to IVF as such, but more likely to be due to the nature of an IVF maternity. It has long been known that a first-born child is typically lower in birth weight than a second-born child. More IVF children are by their very nature *first* born. The average age of an IVF mother is higher. Older maternity has higher risks of placental insufficiency, and thus a risk of poorer fetal growth and subsequent lower birth weight. It is not within the remit of this book to discuss this topic in detail, but the key message here is that many factors recognized as risk factors for an IVF pregnancy are not the result of the process of IVF itself but rather of the couples who need IVF in the first place.

One consideration, however, is the risks associated with higher-order births. The most recent evidence to support the size of this problem studied 42 463 infants born in the USA after ART and compared them with 3 389 098 naturally-conceived children[22]. This showed that the use of assisted reproductive technology accounts for a disproportionate number of low-birth-weight and very-low-birth-weight infants in the USA, in part because of absolute increases in multiple gestations and in part because of higher rates of low birth weight among singleton infants conceived with this texhnology. We all look forward to a day when natural cycle IVF (i.e. that without any hormonal stimulation) results in a single fertilization of a single mature ovum and single embryo replacement. For some couples this will never be an option, but where it is achieved this will dramatically reduce the risks of multiple birth and all that follows from this.

CONGENITAL ANOMALIES

In the early days of IVF a variety of fears arose about the risk of birth defects as a result of this 'unnatural' process. Would congenital malformations occur more often or would these defects occur later? Another line of reasoning[2] was that embryos that were able to survive the artificial circumstances outside the body had to be of a very high quality ('survival of the fittest').

The papers reviewed in Table 2.1 have consistently shown the rate of major malformations of IVF born babies to be in the region of 2%, which is consistent with control populations. The Swedish paper[19] used analysis that included minor anomalies and found the risk ratio for malformations for singleton IVF babies to be 1.25 (1.07–1.46) and multiple births 1.08 (0.93–1.25) in relation to their population as a whole. These show a slightly higher risk than control groups. This is not surprising in the context of older parents with, by inference, older gametes having gone through the stressful and invasive process of IVF to have their child.

One caveat to consider when counselling couples concerning IVF treatments is that it is recognized[23] that 30% of congenital anomalies do not appear until after the newborn period. It is not until very large numbers of children are much older that it will be possible to exclude this. There is a discussion in the concluding chapter about the longer-term risks for IVF children. Two reports[19,24] have suggested a higher incidence of neural tube defects in IVF births. These studies have a weak protocol for drawing such conclusions (the reasons for this are given at the end of Chapter 4).

COMPLICATIONS OF PREMATURITY

Those IVF children born very prematurely are exposed to the same risks of this condition as any other children. These are best summarized by being considered as short-term risks and longer-term risks. Premature babies need to be helped to grow into mature babies in neonatal units. Their attendance in such units is traumatic for their parents and themselves. When counselling parents who are expecting to deliver a premature baby, those risks can be divided into four simple catagories:

(1) *Problems with keeping warm:* these babies have lower body fat and glycogen stores and are at risk of hypothermia and hypoglycemia.
(2) *Problems with breathing and feeding:* using the analogy of a person who has just run up 10 flights of stairs and is then asked to drink a liter of juice, it is easy to understand that breathlessness interferes with drinking milk and thus enteral or parenteral nutrition is sometimes necessary. A knock-on effect is that premature babies are often devoid of the sucking reflex before 32 weeks of gestation. Breathing difficulties due to lung underdevelopment can result in respiratory support being required. This varies from oxygen in the incubator, to continuous positive airways pressure (CPAP), to mechanical ventilation. These therapies have their own risks and complications. Another weakness, both innate and iatrogenic, which interferes with adequate oxygenation is anemia.

(3) *Problems with infections and jaundice:* premature babies are relatively immunoparetic and thus need constant surveillance and treatment for infections they are exposed to. Some of these are from relatively weak commensal organisms and others from more virulent agents. They also need frequent treatment for jaundice, from which they are at higher risk.
(4) *Neurological complications:* depending on gestation, there are risks of long-term neurological sequelae of being born premature. These include conditions such as cerebral palsy, but more subtle conditions such as dyspraxias are now starting to be recognized as more common amongst these children. Visual difficulties are added to these, owing to retinopathy of prematurity. Fortunately, these difficulties are generally treated with laser therapy before long-term complications ensue.

Neurological complications are those that will have long-term overtones for these children and their parents. Within the medical literature there are many reports over and above those reviewed in Table 2.1, which describe complications of being born early from IVF. However, those especially looking at higher-order births are few. A group at the Jones Institute of Reproductive Medicine[25] looked especially at outcomes from IVF twin, triplet and quadruplet IVF pregnancies. This study noted that the incidence of naturally occurring multiple births of higher order was very low[26], and that the incidence of multiple pregnancies has risen ten times since IVF was introduced. The summary of their findings make painful reading to a pediatrician. In 1982–90, 629 IVF pregnancies progressed beyond 20 weeks; there were 115 twins (18.3%), 15 triplets (2.4%) and four quadruplets (0.6%).

There was a high incidence of antenatal complications such as abortions (30.3%, 42% and 20%), premature labor (41.5%, 92.3% and 75%), pregnancy-induced hypertension (17.0%, 38.6% and 50%) and gestational diabetes mellitus (3.1%, 38.5% and 25%) for twins, triplets and quadruplets, respectively. The mean gestational age at delivery was 35.5 ± 3.7, 31.8 ± 2.7 and 31.0 ± 1.7 weeks, respectively. There was also a proportionate progressive increase in neonatal complications. The mean weights were 2473 ± 745, 1666 ± 441 and 1414 ± 368 g, respectively. Twins (22.7%), 64.1% of triplets and 75% of quadruplets needed admission to the neonatal intensive care unit and remained for an average of 12.0 ± 2.3, 17.4 ± 14.0 and 57.8 ± 17.9 days, respectively. There was no difference in the mean Apgar scores or the incidence of congenital malformations in the three groups. The corrected perinatal mortality rates were 38.5, 0.0 and 0.0 per 1000 live births, respectively. This paper[27] brings out the reality of problems to be anticipated by couples considering IVF, so desperate to have children as to request more than one embryo to be replaced. The morbidity and mortality brought about by this phenomenon was recognized quite early[27] in the UK. A study in 1993[28] reported that 8% of babies from assisted conception were born with a birth weight of <1500 g versus 1% of those conceived naturally. It is also clear from the Human Fertilisation and Embryology Authority data analysis[29] that the effect of replacing three embryos as opposed to two is not an increase in *overall* pregnancy rate but merely an increase in the rate of triplet pregnancies and births. This is regardless of the maternal age. Any counsellor or prospective parent reading this book should give this fact careful consideration.

There is little further work specifically looking at complications of IVF-conceived premature infants, but there are two which investigated the morbidity specifically due to retinopathy of prematurity (ROP)[29,30]. Both these British studies advised that ROP appeared to present more frequently and more severely in this group of premature babies. This therefore should be a factor taken into account by ophthalmic surgeons when screening for ROP in neonatal units.

In summary, the outcomes for premature babies relate to gestation at birth. IVF infants are at higher risk of being born early, although this appears to be a reducing trend. Infants with extremely low birth weight (those born at < 1000 g) continue to do badly. Although interventions such as prophylactic antenatal steroids[31] or exogenous surfactants[32] have improved certain outcomes, the overall prognosis is poor. In North America a multicenter cohort study of infants with extremely low birth weight found that less than two-thirds of those admitted to intensive care survived to hospital discharge. A quarter of surviving children, assessed at 18–24 months post-term, had an abnormal neurological examination, and about one-third had evidence of significant neurological developmental delay[33]. In the UK and Eire, the EPICure Study group evaluated the outcome for infants born before 26 weeks' gestation. The overall survival of infants admitted to intensive care was 39%[34]. When assessed at a mean age of 30 months post-term, about half the children had a disability, and about half of these met the predefined criteria for severe disability[35].

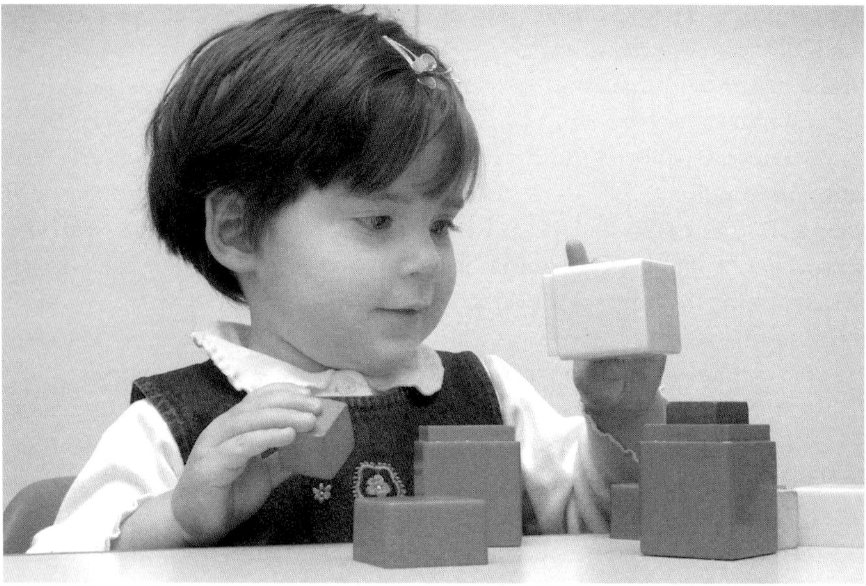

Figure 2.1 Elâ Iona Sutcliffe performing one item of the Griffiths scales of mental development for children 0–2 years of age

BEYOND THE NEONATAL PERIOD

Research has focused on certain core outcomes, the main ones being neurodevelopment. A Swedish study[36] investigated 99 IVF children of mean age 62 months. No control group was assessed. All were assessed using the Griffiths scales of mental development (Figure 2.1) and the Achenbach's Child Behavior Checklist (CBCL). In comparison with population norms, behavior and cognitive development were considered to be normal. An Australian study[37] investigated 314 IVF children, which were case matched with 150 control children. The only matching that was not done was for triplets. This seminal paper, written in 1996, suggested that IVF status was not a significant independent factor for physical outcome, including malformation rates (although the caveat for this is that this study was far too weak for this to be concluded positively), nor for days of hospitalization after discharge, and operations. Children were of 2 years of age (mean) and seemed to be growing adequately. The only other reservation about the findings was the response rate of those requested to be seen in the study, which was only 81% in the IVF group, which may allow for some bias from non-attendees. In a UK study[38] a cohort of

278 children, conceived by IVF after the transfer of three fresh embryos, were followed for 4 years and were assessed for neonatal conditions, minor anomalies, major congenital anomalies, cerebral palsy and other disabilities; control children were matched appropriately. Two children, born from multiple births, had cerebral palsy, and the mean developmental quotient in the IVF group was 116 (119 in the IVF singleton children, 106 in those with multiple birth, at a mean age of 2 years). The outcome was predictably less satisfactory for children from premature births. Notably the paper concluded that a reduction of multiple pregnancies, by limiting the transfer of embryos to two instead of three, remains a high priority. The developmental quotients in this particular study were assessed by the Griffiths neurodevelopmental testing system. A French study[39] investigated the outcome of 422 children, aged 6–13 years, conceived by IVF. Although the aims of the study were laudable, the methods by which the children were assessed were too weak to render the study of much meaning. These families were all contacted by telephone and by questionnaire, and developmental well-being was inferred by the rank of the child in their class, at the educational institute they were attending, at the time. This would be effectively meaningless if it did not take into account the education being given at the particular school, which the child had been attending from an early age. However, this study is the one that has taken children to the oldest age to date. As far as can be concluded, the rates of malformation did not seem to be any different from normal, and school performance was good on the whole. Rather worryingly, the study reported that 58% of parents of children aged 6–10 years had not informed their children about the IVF, nor had 34% of the children aged 11–13 years been told.

A study investigated the possibility of radiological abnormalities in children born as a result of assisted conception[40]. Apart from the known complications related to prematurity, which affect all premature babies, these children were not thought to have any specific radiological features distinguishing them from other children. Another study was performed[41], which looked at 95 infants born as a result of IVF and compared them with 79 naturally conceived control children, between the ages of 4 and 12 months, to investigate whether infants conceived using IVF were utilizing health-care resources more often after the neonatal period. The study concluded that, in the medium term, IVF infants did not appear to have an increased number of medical problems or to overutilize health-care resources during the remainder of their first year of life.

Finally, the subject of the incidence of cancer in children born after IVF was investigated by Bruinsma and colleagues[42], using a record-linkage cohort design. The study involved all conceptions using assisted reproductive technologies between 1979 and 1995, in the state of Victoria, Australia. This important study included only 5249 births. To the uninformed reader this may seem a large number but for cancer, which is rare, larger numbers would ideally be required. The conclusion was that, during the mean follow-up period of 3 years and 9 months, there was a slightly higher number of cases than would be predicted in this group; 4.33 cases of cancer were expected and 6 were observed. In view of the 'relatively' small sample size, this does not give any cause for concern. The theoretical reasons for children from IVF conceptions possibly being at higher risk of getting cancer are discussed in Chapter 6. Other studies that considered childhood cancer as a possible outcome have not been referred to, because they had even fewer participants.

CONCLUSIONS

Children conceived after IVF are generally healthy and developmentally normal, the exception being those born prematurely (which is a very high risk) and those born from multiple births. In these circumstances they will be at higher risk of complications related to prematurity and exceptional risk, within that group, of retinopathy of prematurity.

Much consideration has been given to whether there might be an impact on family relationships, but to date no definitive evidence has been provided to support the suggestion that their family relationships are in some way distorted. There is inadequate evidence, even 23 years after Louise Brown was born, that in the longer term these children will not be at risk of other problems, such as cancer or infertility. However, as far as the data have been forthcoming, there is a generally reassuring picture.

REFERENCES

1. Snowden R, Snowden E. Families created through donor insemination. In Daniels K, Haimes E, (eds.) *Donor Insemination*. Cambridge: Cambridge University Press, 1998:33–52
2. Van Balen F. Development of IVF children. *Dev Rev* 1998;18:30–46
3. McWhinnie A. Outcome for families created by assisted conception programmes. *J Assist Reprod Genet* 1996;13:363–5
4. Colpin H, Demyttenaere K, Vandemeulebroecke L. New reproductive technology and the family: the parent–child relationship following *in vitro* fertilization. *J Child Psychol Psychiatry* 1995;36:1429–41

5. Mushin D, Spensley J, Barreda-Hanson M. Children of IVF. *Clin Obstet Gynaecol* 1985;12:865–76
6. Pullan-Watkins K. *Reference Books on Family Issues:* vol. 2. *Parent–Child Attachment: a Guide to Research.* Garland Reference Library on Social Science 388. New York: Garland, 1987
7. Golombok R, Cook R, Bish A, Moray C. Families created by the new reproductive technologies: quality of parenting and social and emotional development of the children. *Child Dev* 1995;66:285–98
8. Cook R, Bradley S, Golombok S. A preliminary study of parental stress and child behaviour in families with twins conceived by *in vitro* fertilization. *Hum Reprod* 1998;13:3244–6
9. McWhinnie A. Should offspring from donated gametes continue to be denied knowledge of their origins and antecedents? *Hum Rep* 2001;5:807–17
10. Roegiers L. Fecondation *in vitro*, cadeua ou fardeau? Quelques considerations systemiques et ethiques sur la souffrance du couple infertile et la place de l'enfant qui se fait longtemps attendre. *Therapie Familiale* 1992;13:41–54
11. Colpin H. Parents and children of reproductive technology: chances and risks for their well-being. *Community Alternatives: Int J Fam Care* 1994;6:49–71
12. Raoul-Duval A, Bertrand-Servais M, Frydman R. Comparative prospective study of the psychological development of children born by *in vitro* fertilization and their mothers. *J Psychosom Obstet Gynaecol* 1993;14:117–26
13. Hahn CS, DiPietro JA. *In vitro* fertilization and the family: quality of parenting, family functioning, and child psychosocial adjustment. *Dev Psychol* 2001;37:37–48
14. Sutcliffe AG. Intracytoplasmic sperm injection and other aspects of new reproductive technologies. *Arch Dis Child* 2000;83:98–101
15. Rufat P, Dehan M, Olivennes F, *et al.* Task force on the outcome of pregnancies and children conceived by *in vitro* fertilization (France: 1987 to 1989). *Fertil Steril* 1994;2:324–30
16. Dhont M, De Sutter P, Ruyssinck G, *et al.* Perinatal outcome of pregnancies after assisted reproduction: a case–control study. *Am J Obstet Gynecol* 1999;3:688–95
17. FIVNAT. Pregnancies and births resulting from *in vitro* fertilization: French national registry, analysis of data 1986 to 1990. *Fertil Steril* 1995;4:746–56
18. Westergaard HB, Tranberg Johansen AM, Erb K, Nyboe Andersen A. Danish National IVF Registry 1994 and 1995. Treatment, pregnancy outcome and complications during pregnancy. *Acta Obstet Gynecol Scand* 2000;79:384–9
19. Bergh T, Ericson A, Hillensjo T, *et al.* Deliveries and children born after *in-vitro* fertilisation in Sweden 1982–95: a retrospective cohort study. *Lancet* 1999;354: 1579–85
20. Friedler S, Mashiach S, Laufer N. Births in Israel resulting from *in-vitro* fertilization/embryo transfer, 1982–1989: National Registry of Israeli Association for Fertility Research. *Hum Reprod* 1992;8:1159–63
21. MRC Working party on children conceived by *in vitro* fertilization. Births in Great Britain resulting from assisted conception, 1978–87. *Br Med J* 1990;300: 1229–3
22. Schieve LA, Meikle SF, Ferre C, *et al.* Low and very low birth weight in infants conceived with use of assisted reproductive technology. *N Engl J Med* 2002;346:731–7
23. EUROCAT Central Registry Department of Epidemiology. *Surveillance of Congenital Abnormalities 1980–1988*. Brussels: Eurocat Central Registry, 1991
24. Lancaster PA. Health registers for congenital malformations and *in vitro* fertilization. *Clin Reprod Fertil* 1986;4:27–37

25. Seoud O. Outcome of twin, triplet, and quadruplet *in vitro* fertilisation pregnancies: the Norfolk experience of IVF twins. *Fertil Steril* 1992;57:825–34
26. Schnorr JA, Doviak MJ, Muasher SJ, Jones HW Jr. Impact of a cryopreservation program on the multiple pregnancy rate associated with assisted reproductive technologies. *Fertil Steril* 2001;75:147–51
27. Levene MI, Wild J, Steer P. Higher multiple births and the modern management of infertility in Britain. The British Association of Perinatal Medicine. *Br J Obstet Gynaecol* 1992;99:607–13
28. McFaul PB, Patel N, Mills J. An audit of the obstetric outcome of 148 consecutive pregnancies from assisted conception: implications for neonatal services. *Br J Obstet Gynaecol* 1993;100:820–5
29. Watts P, Adams GG. *In vitro* fertilisation and stage 3 retinopathy of prematurity. *Eye* 2000;14:330–3
30. McKibbin M, Booth AP, Dabbs TR. *In vitro* fertilisation and stage 3 retinopathy of prematurity. *Eye* 2001;15:363–4
31. Crowley P. Prophylactic corticosteroids for preterm birth. *Cochrane Database Syst Rev* 2000;2:CD000065
32. Schwartz RM, Luby AM, Scanlon JW, Kellogg RJ. Effect of surfactant on morbidity, mortality and resource use in newborn infants weighing 500 to 1500g. *N Engl J Med* 1994;330:1476–80
33. Vohr BR, Wright LL, Dusick AM, *et al.* Neurodevelopmental and functional outcomes of extremely low birth weight infants in National Institute of Child Health and Human Development Neonatal Research Network, 1993–1994. *Pediatrics* 2000; 105:1216–26
34. Costloe K, Hennessy E, Gibson AT, Marlow N, Wilkinson AR. The EPICure study: outcomes to discharge from hospital infants born at the threshold of viability. *Pediatrics* 2000;106:659–71
35. Wood NS, Marlow N, Costloe K, Gibson AT, Wilkinson AR. Neurologic and developmental disability after extremely preterm birth. EPICure Study Group. *N Engl J Med* 2000;343:378–84
36. Cederblad M, Friberg B, Ploman F, *et al.* Intelligence and behaviour in children born after *in-vitro* fertilization treatment. *Hum Reprod* 1996;11:2052–7
37. Saunders K, Spensley J, Munro J, Halasz G. Growth and physical outcome of children conceived by *in vitro* fertilization. *Pediatrics* 1996;97:688–92
38. D'Souza SW, Rivlin E, Cadman J, Richards B, Buck P, Lieberman BA. Children conceived by *in vitro* fertilisation after fresh embryo transfer. *Arch Dis Child Fetal Neonatal Ed* 1997;76:F70–4
39. Olivennes F, Kerbrat V, Rufat P, *et al.* Follow-up of a cohort of 422 children aged 6 to 13 years conceived by *in vitro* fertilization. *Fertil Steril* 1997;67:284–9
40. Leighton DM. Radiological abnormalities in children born as a result of assisted conception. *Aust Radiol* 1995;39:237–42
41. Leslie GI, Gibson FL, McMahon C, *et al.* Infants conceived using *in-vitro* fertilization do not over-utilize health care resources after the neonatal period. *Hum Reprod* 1998;13:2055–9
42. Bruinsma F, Venn A, Lancaster P, *et al.* Incidence of cancer in children born after *in-vitro* fertilization. *Hum Reprod* 2000;15:604–7

3

Children born after embryo cryopreservation

'The only thing constant in life is change'

Francois de la Rochefoucauld

INTRODUCTION

I was privileged to be the first person to study neurodevelopmental outcome in children from embryos that had been frozen. It was via this study that my interest in the subject of assisted reproductive therapies and their outcome arose. At a press presentation of the work an article was written in a regional newspaper. Reflecting on the finding that the children I studied were of above average intelligence, the article was entitled 'sharp little frosties'. Sadly this reflects the superficiality and sensationalist way in which this subject is often dealt with by the lay press.

Cryopreserved human embryos, later thawed then transferred into women were first described as part of an *in vitro* fertilization (IVF) program by Trounson and Mohr[1]. Cryopreservation of embryos plays an important role in IVF with the use of superovulation regimens and advances in embryo culture and cryopreservation techniques. Cryopreservation of oocytes is now possible and this, along with other developments, may ultimately reduce the need for cryopreservation of embryos. Cryopreservation of embryos has certain advantages; for example, greater usage can be made of a high oocyte yield after treatment with gonadotropin releasing hormone. Since only two embryos are transferred (to reduce the frequency of multiple births), the remaining embryos could be cryopreserved and used later. Some women, after undergoing induction of ovulation, develop ovarian

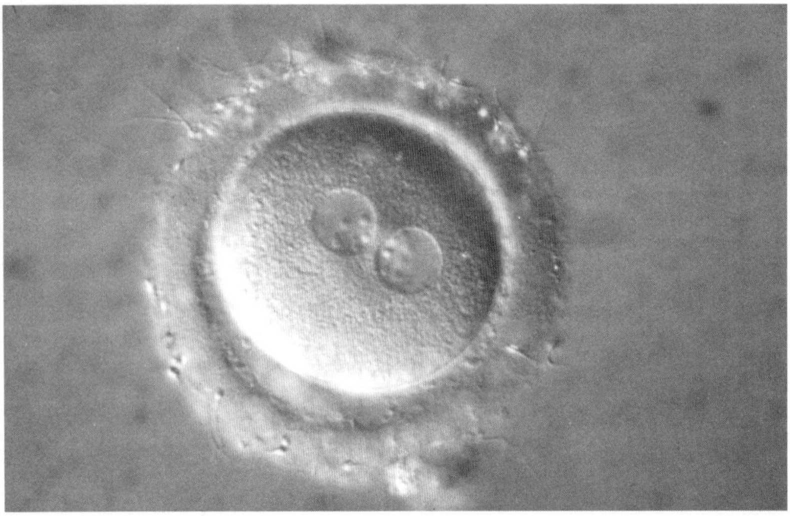

Figure 3.1 A human pronucleate embryo at the developmental stage where cryopreservation is performed

hyperstimulation syndrome, a condition characterized by massive ovarian enlargement and shifts in body fluids leading to ascites and hydrothorax. In such women, IVF can be carried out after recovery from the condition using cryopreserved/thawed embryos. Satisfactory survival rates in human embryos replaced at the pronucleate stage (Figure 3.1) have been reported at the IVF unit where my study was undertaken[2].

LABORATORY TECHNIQUES FOR EMBRYO FREEZING

Cryopreservation techniques for human embryos have evolved considerably since the first pregnancy was achieved in 1983 following the transfer of an eight-cell embryo[1]. The first birth was reported in 1985[3], following the transfer of a frozen–thawed blastocyst using glycerol as the cryoprotectant. In recent years embryos have been more commonly frozen at the pronucleate or early cleavage stages using the method described by Lassalle and colleagues 1985[4], using propanediol and sucrose (Figures 3.2 and 3.3).

Cryoprotectants

During cryopreservation, all chemical reactions within cells should be suspended. Human embryos are stored under liquid nitrogen at –190 °C, a

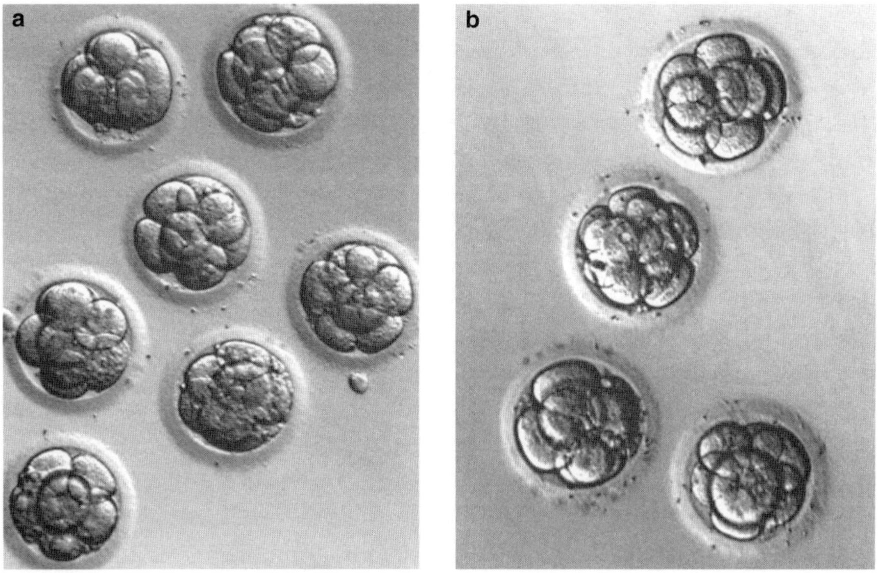

Figure 3.2 (a) Seven apparently healthy conceptuses shown before freezing on day 3 after harvest. (b) Four of the pre-embryos were thawed 122 days later; all survived. Unfortunately, no pregnancy was established in the 38-year-old woman who produced these conceptuses. Figures reproduced with kind permission of Lucinda L. Veeck, MLT, hDSc, Cornell University Medical College, New York, USA

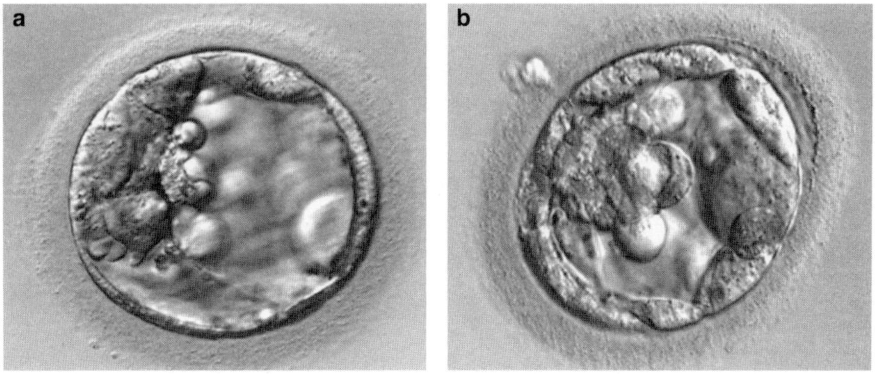

Figure 3.3 Early blastocysts, frozen for 3 years in 10% gycerol, shown just after thawing. Despite a relatively normal appearance, their transfer to a 42-year-old woman failed to result in pregnancy. Figures reproduced with kind permission of Lucinda L. Veeck, MLT, hDSc, Cornell University Medical College, New York, USA

temperature at which the only deterioration is likely to be due to background ionizing radiation, which would take hundreds of years to do significant damage[4]. Damage does occur as a result of cryopreservation – not during the storage phase, but during the cooling or thawing process. Damage generally occurs as a result of ice crystal formation within the cells, or changes in osmotic pressure as a result of water loss from the cell. Slow cooling limits both these types of damage, as does the use of cryoprotectants, such as propanediol, dimethylsulfoxide (DMSO) or glycerol. Slow cooling reduces the rate of water loss from the cell, and the consequent increase in salt concentration which results from ice crystal formation in the surrounding medium. Cryoprotectants also act in this way and in addition help to reduce the risk of intracellular ice formation. The current most popular technique for cryopreservation of pronucleate and early cleavage stage embryos utilizes propanediol, which penetrates the cells rapidly, in combination with sucrose, which causes water to leave the cells[5]. This has almost entirely replaced the use of DMSO, a far more toxic substance that required a longer, more complicated protocol and gave disappointing results.

KNOWN OUTCOMES

A relatively recent study[6], which compared the birth characteristics and perinatal outcome in infants from cryopreserved embryos with those after fresh embryo transfer, has shown that the mean gestational age and birth weight were not significantly different between the groups. There was no difference in perinatal mortality rates and the incidence of major congenital anomalies was significantly lower in the cryopreserved than in the fresh embryo group.

Previous studies on the obstetric outcome in IVF have reported a higher incidence of multiple pregnancies, preterm delivery, Cesarean section and fetal growth restriction[7–9]. There are similarities between these findings and those reported in women after transfer of cryopreserved embryos[10]. In the British study described below, the outcome of a group of children from cryopreserved embryos was compared with that of normally conceived children.

The British study

This study was completed between August 1993 and September 1994 while I was working at the University of Manchester, and has formed the basis of two scientific papers[11,12] with findings also presented at scientific meetings. Out of an original group of 111 children still living in the north-west region of England, 91 children were seen by me and compared with 83 naturally conceived control children. The results are presented herein.

In the cryopreserved embryo group (n = 91) there were 68 singletons, with the remaining 23 children from multiple births, including 20 twin and three triplet children. The controls (n = 83) consisted of 81 singleton and two twin children. The demographic data for these two groups of children are shown in Table 3.1. The lower birth weight ($p < 0.001$) in the cryopreserved group reflected a higher proportion of preterm births. In the cryopreserved embryo group, ten (12.7%) of 79 births were preterm (< 37 weeks' gestational age) as compared with six (7.3%) of 82 births in the control group ($p < 0.01$). There was a higher proportion of preterm births from multiple pregnancies: three (27.3%) of 11 as compared with seven (10.3%) of 68 singleton pregnancies from cryopreserved embryos ($p < 0.01$). A comparison of the proportion of children born by Cesarean section and vaginal delivery showed that a higher proportion of the former were from the cryopreserved embryo group as compared with controls (52% vs. 13%, $p < 0.001$, Table 3.1).

Clinical assessment

The neurological conditions found on clinical examination included squints and conductive hearing loss (Table 3.2). There was one child with Down syndrome in the cryopreserved embryo group. This child was included in the assessment and analysis in order to provide the most objective comparison of this population.

Griffiths scales of mental development

The two groups were assessed at a similar chronological age not corrected for preterm birth. Correction was thought likely to mask any developmental problems arising and thus weaken the clinical usefulness of such an assessment. Griffiths scales are designed to be used without correction for gestational age. The mean mental age was higher (by 5.29 months) in the control group as compared with the cryopreserved embryo group, and there was an associated increase in the mean Griffiths quotient, which did not reach statistical significance. With respect to the sub-quotients for locomotor, personal/social, hearing and speech, eye–hand co-ordination and performance, the only significant difference was in hearing and speech,

Table 3.1 Demographic details and early life of infants from cryopreserved embryos and control infants. Where applicable, results are mean ± SD

	Cryopreserved embryos			
	Singleton ($n = 68$)	*Multiple births* ($n = 23$)	*Total* ($n = 91$)	*Controls* ($n = 83$)
Birth weight (g)	$3282.6 \pm 672.8^{+++}$	2649.7 ± 649.2	$3122.6 \pm 721.4^{***}$	3538.4 ± 553.4
Gestational age (weeks)	$38.59 \pm 2.36^{++}$	37.09 ± 1.62	$38.38 \pm 2.33^{***}$	39.67 ± 1.96
Mode of delivery				
vaginal	34	10	44	72
Cesarean section	34	13	47^{***}	11
SCBU admissions	11	2	13	5
Hyaline membrane disease	1	0	1	0
Transient tachypnea	2	1	3	2
Hypothermia (< 36°C)	4	0	4	0
Failure to feed	1	1	2	1
Vomiting	1	0	1	0
Small for gestational age	2	0	2	2
Boys	39	11	50	40
Girls	29	12	41	43
Social class of father				
0 (unemployed)			1 (1.1%)	2 (2.4%)
1			21 (23.1%)	29 (34.9%)
2			31 (34.1%)	34 (41.0%)
3			28 (30.8%)	16 (19.3%)
> 4			10 (11.0%)	2 (2.4%)

SCBU, special care baby unit

Total (cryopreserved embryo) vs. controls: $^{***}p < 0.001$; singleton (cryopreserved embryo) vs. multiple births (cryopreserved embryo): $^{+++}p < 0.001$, $^{++}p < 0.01$

Table 3.2 Outcomes of clinical assessment

	Cryopreserved embryos			
	Singleton (*n* = 68)	*Multiple births* (*n* = 23)	*Total* (*n* = 91)	*Controls* (*n* = 83)
Squint	3	0	3	6
Conductive hearing loss	4	0	4	9
Down syndrome	1	0	1	0

although the results in both groups were within the normal range (Table 3.3). In the cryopreserved embryo group the Griffiths quotient and the subquotients were compared in children from the singleton and the multiple birth subgroups, but none was significantly different. The mean mental age in these subgroups was similar.

Minor and major congenital anomalies

Table 3.4 shows the types of minor and major congenital anomalies which occurred in relatively small numbers in the two groups of children. Some children had more than one recordable minor congenital anomaly. Hemangiomas (strawberry nevi) were noted more frequently than the remaining minor congenital anomalies in both groups of children. There were 21 children who had one or two hemangiomas about 1 cm in width. An ear defect recorded in three children (all in the cryopreserved embryo group) appeared to be due to a fibrocartilaginous defect that altered the normal configuration of the pinna, but hearing was not adversely affected. A comparison of the proportion of children with minor congenital anomalies in the 'total' group from cryopreserved embryos with that in controls showed that they were statistically similar: 31.9% and 21.7%, respectively (Table 3.4).

The proportion of children with a major congenital anomaly in the total group from cryopreserved embryos was similar to that in controls: 3.3% and 2.4%, respectively (Table 3.4). The major congenital anomalies were Down syndrome, Beckwith–Wiedemann syndrome and hypophosphatemic rickets in children from cryopreserved embryos. Down syndrome (47,XY+21) was diagnosed shortly after birth, and was thought to be due to a non-disjunction defect. There was associated congenital heart disease with an atrial septal defect. The child with Beckwith–Wiedemann syndrome had a history of

Table 3.3 Griffiths scales of mental development, mean scores ± SD

	Cryopreserved embryos			
	Singleton ($n = 68$)	*Multiple births* ($n = 23$)	*Total* ($n = 91$)	*Controls* ($n = 83$)
Chronological age (months)	24.39 ± 12.13	27.15 ± 14.61	25.08 ± 12.86	29.19 ± 14.65
Griffiths quotient	105.04 ± 14.47	107.61 ± 10.12	105.69 ± 13.55	108.18 ± 9.80
Mental age (months)	25.97 ± 14.21	29.13 ± 16.57	26.77 ± 14.91	32.06 ± 17.09*
Sub-quotients				
locomotor	104.54 ± 17.95	108.52 ± 13.05	105.55 ± 16.93	104.10 ± 11.73
personal/social	108.78 ± 17.91	111.00 ± 10.76	109.34 ± 16.43	109.18 ± 12.12
hearing and speech	106.18 ± 21.24	108.04 ± 13.14	106.65 ± 19.53	112.33 ± 13.87*
eye–hand co-ordination	100.85 ± 14.53	105.26 ± 9.46	101.97 ± 19.53	106.20 ± 15.11
performance	105.01 ± 16.68	106.96 ± 12.50	105.51 ± 15.75	108.40 ± 15.32

Cryopreserved embryo (total) vs. controls: $^*p < 0.05$

Table 3.4 Major and minor congenital anomalies in children from cryopreserved embryos and controls

	Study children			*Control children*		
	Singleton (*n* = 68)	*Multiple births* (*n* = 23)	*Total* (*n* = 91)	*Singleton* (*n* = 81)	*Multiple births* (*n* = 2)	*Total* (*n* = 83)
Ear defect	3	0	3	0	0	0
Hammer toe	1	0	1	0	0	0
Tongue tie	1	0	1	0	0	0
Plagiocephaly	0	1	1	0	0	0
Pectus excavatum	0	0	0	1	0	1
Hypermetropia	0	0	0	1	0	1
Web toes	2	0	2	1	0	1
Sacral dimple	0	0	0	2	0	2
Laryngeal stridor	1	1	2	0	0	0
Phimosis	0	0	0	1	0	1
Undescended testes	1	0	1	0	0	0
Talipes equinovarus	1	2	3	0	0	0
Pigmented nevus	1	1	2	5	0	5
Hemangioma	10	4	14	7	0	7
Umbilical hernia	2	0	2	0	0	0
Single palmar crease	1	0	1	0	0	0
Total minor	24	9	33	18	0	18
Hydronephrosis	0	0	0	1	0	1
Gastroschisis	0	0	0	1	0	1
Down syndrome	1	0	1	0	0	0
Beckwith–Wiedemann syndome	1	0	1	0	0	0
Hypophosphatemic rickets	0	1	1	0	0	0
Total major	2	1	3	2	0	2
No. of children with minor anomaly	22	7	29	18	0	18
% with minor	32.4	30.4	31.9	22.2	(–)	21.7
No. of children with major anomaly	2	1	3	2	0	2
% with major	2.9	4.3	3.3	2.5	(–)	2.4

transient neonatal hypoglycemia due to hyperinsulinemia, parallel skin creases in both ear lobes, exomphalos and macroglossia, which regressed as the child grew older. Hypophosphatemic rickets, diagnosed in the first year, was characterized by low plasma phosphate and radiographic changes in the long bones. Hydronephrosis and gastroschisis were diagnosed in the control

Table 3.5 Odds ratio plus 95% confidence intervals of a minor congenital anomaly and a major congenital anomaly in children from cryopreserved embryos (C) as compared with normally conceived children as controls (N)

	Singleton pregnancies (N = 81, C = 68)	*Multiple pregnancies* (N = 2, C = 23)	*All pregnancies* (N = 83, C = 91)
Minor congenital anomaly	1.7 (0.8–3.5)	—	1.7 (0.8–3.3)
Major congenital anomaly	1.2 (0.2–8.7)	—	1.4 (0.2–8.5)

Note: There were no congenital abnormalities recorded in the normally conceived multiple pregnancies

children during the neonatal period. The odds ratio (and 95% confidence intervals) of minor congenital anomalies and major congenital anomalies in children from cryopreserved embryos compared with controls is shown in Table 3.5. There was no family history of similar minor congenital anomalies or of major congenital anomalies nor were congenital anomalies related to maternal education or alcohol intake during pregnancy or to maternal occupation.

Effect of minor congenital anomalies and major congenital anomalies on developmental indices (Griffiths scales of mental development)

Table 3.6 shows that the mean Griffiths quotient (GQ) was greater than the standard 100 in children with minor congenital anomalies, and major congenital anomalies, *and* in children without an abnormality, both in the cryopreserved embryo group and in controls. A comparison of the mean GQ in these subgroups of children, with or without a congenital abnormality, showed that there was no significant difference in the cryopreserved embryo group.

In the controls the mean GQ was significantly higher in children with minor congenital anomalies and major congenital anomalies than in children without an abnormality. In the cryopreserved embryo group and in controls the mean Griffiths sub-quotient for locomotor, personal/social, hearing and speech, eye–hand co-ordination, performance and practical reasoning were compared. There were significant differences in personal/social and eye–hand co-ordination subquotients when children with minor congenital anomalies and major congenital anomalies were compared with

Table 3.6 Association between minor congenital anomaly and the Griffiths quotient (mean ± SD)

	Cases			*Controls*		
	With anomaly ($n = 32$)	*Without anomaly* ($n = 59$)	*Total* ($n = 91$)	*With anomaly* ($n = 20$)	*Without anomaly* ($n = 63$)	*Total* ($n = 83$)
Chronological age (months)	24.04 ± 13.32	25.65 ± 12.56	25.08 ± 12.86	29.33 ± 15.51	29.15 ± 14.37	29.19 ± 14.65
Mental age (months)	24.78 ± 14.67	27.85 ± 14.93	26.77 ± 14.91	33.75 ± 18.68	31.52 ± 16.52	32.06 ± 17.09
Griffiths quotient	103.00 ± 13.79	107.15 ± 13.19	105.69 ± 13.55	$113.20^{*} \pm 11.17$	106.59 ± 8.75	108.18 ± 9.80
Sub-quotients						
locomotor	103.00 ± 17.90	106.93 ± 16.22	105.55 ± 16.93	107.20 ± 14.94	103.11 ± 10.31	104.10 ± 11.73
personal/social	105.72 ± 17.52	111.31 ± 15.46	109.34 ± 16.43	$115.60^{**} \pm 13.28$	107.14 ± 10.97	109.18 ± 12.12
hearing and speech	103.66 ± 20.16	108.27 ± 18.98	106.65 ± 19.53	116.90 ± 13.81	110.87 ± 13.57	112.33 ± 13.87
eye–hand co-ordination	99.69 ± 13.79	103.20 ± 13.28	101.97 ± 13.56	$114.45^{**} \pm 15.62$	103.59 ± 13.97	106.20 ± 15.11
performance	103.00 ± 14.26	106.86 ± 16.34	105.51 ± 15.75	110.20 ± 13.82	107.83 ± 15.73	108.40 ± 15.32
practical reasoning	106.93 ± 13.10	110.83 ± 19.84	109.53 ± 17.97	116.79 ± 17.03	110.63 ± 12.18	112.29 ± 13.92

Congenital abnormality = minor + major congenital anomaly
Levels of significance: congenital abnormality vs. without abnormality: $^{*}p < 0.05$; $^{**}p < 0.01$

those without such congenital abnormalities in the control group but not in the cryopreserved embryo group.

In the total group of children from cryopreserved embryos, or controls, there were no significant differences in the mean GQ or the mean Griffiths subquotient values (Table 3.6).

Comments

These results provided the first evidence that children born from frozen embryos were developmentally normal and had similar congenital abnormality rates to control, normally conceived children. There were limitations regarding the choice of control children in this study. It proved impossible to match control children by parental age, parity, multiplicity of pregnancy or history of infertility – all factors possibly predictive of increased obstetric risk[12–15]. IVF mothers tend to be older than average, their infertility might indicate genetic or other medical disorders and they have a higher incidence of multiple pregnancy, Cesarean section and preterm births[7–9].

However, although numbers were not large, children from cryopreserved embryos did not have an increased rate of neurological abnormality or major disability such as cerebral palsy at follow-up, despite a higher incidence of preterm births. Such increased risks have been previously reported in children with low birth weight including results from a geographically defined population[16]. An increased risk of squints and conductive deafness has also been reported in children with low birth weight[17], and squints have been reported in children conceived by IVF[8]. In the present study the frequency of squints and conductive hearing loss in the cryopreserved embryo group and in controls was similar. It seems unlikely that the procedures used in cryopreservation or thawing of embryos predispose to the development of squints or conductive hearing loss.

The results, even including the child with Down syndrome, are concordant with previous studies on the development of children conceived by IVF using fresh embryos[18–20]. The mean GQ in the cryopreserved embryo group and in controls was above the standard 100. It may be that the family background in these two groups of children placed them at a developmental advantage. It may also reflect the fact that the scales were last standardized 20 years before. Developmental attainment appears to be occurring at earlier ages with modern child rearing, which includes rising nutritional status and greater access to education. In the new infant scales, which became available in 1996, during the restandardization infants given a new score of 100 were scoring a mean of 108 on the old scales[21].

The mode of conception using normal conceptions as the comparison did not significantly affect mean mental age in children from cryopreserved embryos. The small reduction in the GQ compared with controls was due to the cases being a mean of 4 months younger than controls. In these circumstances the statistically significant differences between the mental age are irrelevant and in the hearing and speech sub-quotients are of no practical importance. It is noteworthy that, in the cryopreserved embryo group, children from multiple births and singleton birth showed comparable performance for a range of sub-quotients; as a consequence their mean GQs were statistically similar (Table 3.3).

By contrast, in a previous study of children conceived by IVF (largely fresh embryo transfer), twin and triplet children performed less well than singletons when tested at a similar chronological age using the Griffiths scales of mental development[22].

The proportion of children from cryopreserved embryos with major congenital anomalies, 3.3%, is similar to that reported by the Medical Research Council (MRC) Working Party on Children Conceived by *In Vitro* Fertilisation[8]. IVF pregnancies resulting from the transfer of cryopreserved–thawed embryos or fresh embryos appear to be associated with higher perinatal mortality rates than the UK national average. This difference has been largely attributed to an increase in multiple pregnancies and preterm births after assisted conception rather than to other factors such as an overall increase in congenital anomaly rate. In the MRC survey analyzing 1581 live born/stillborn children, the number of cases of children with specific types of anomaly was small, but there appeared to be an excess of conditions affecting the central nervous system. Some rare medical disorders were reported in the survey including craniostenosis, Russell–Silver syndrome, osteogenesis imperfecta, persistent cloaca, absent genitalia, partial albinism and extensive areas of depigmentation. None of these conditions were seen in our children from cryopreserved embryos, but there was a case of Beckwith–Wiedemann syndrome and one of hypophosphatemic rickets, conditions not reported in the MRC survey.

Most children with minor congenital anomalies in this study had hemangiomas or pigmented nevi, and the frequency of such anomalies was statistically similar in the cryopreserved embryo group and controls (Table 3.4).

Minor congenital anomalies have not received much attention when surveys of the outcome of IVF pregnancies have been reported. However, in a prospective study of children conceived by IVF, Morin and associates[19] looked for more than 130 major and minor anomalies and found major anomalies in two children (a frequency of 2.4%): one with a non-patent auditory canal, hearing loss and microtia and the other with a thoracic meningomyelocele and hypoplasia of the scrotum. Morin and colleagues also reported an increased frequency of two minor congenital anomalies, significantly higher than controls: a Darwinian point and a high arched palate. These conditions were not seen in the study children.

In the present analysis the relative risk was determined of major congenital abnormalities and minor congenital anomalies in the children from cryopreserved embryos in relation to controls (Table 3.4). The results suggest that the risks in the study group may not be higher than in the controls. There are, however, possible risks associated with the technique of IVF and embryo transfer, which might increase the probability of birth defects. Biggers[23] suggested a likely increase due to an increase in the level of chromosomal aberrations, fertilization with abnormal spermatozoa, induction of point mutations, or the actions of physical and chemical teratogens. He drew attention to an increase in the level of trisomy among abortuses in women who had been induced to ovulate, a high incidence of chromosomal aberrations occurring as a result of superovulation in animal experiments and an increase in triploidy when ova were exposed to spermatozoa in high concentrations. The present study did not identify a family history of congenital abnormalities, with rates in the cryopreserved embryo group being similar to those in controls. There was no association with maternal medication, alcohol intake or occupation.

Chromosomal aberrations found in human embryos include monosomies and trisomies[23] and these embryos may not be distinguished morphologically from those with normal chromosomes[24]. The presence of such abnormal chromosomes may not prevent early embryonic development, but few fetuses are capable of progressing to term, so they are eliminated as spontaneous abortions. Down syndrome and other chromosomal abnormalities have been reported in a survey of births resulting from IVF[8]. The proportion of births from transfer of cryopreserved embryos was not clearly specified in that survey.

Rizk and co-workers[25] reported Edward syndrome (trisomy 18) in a fetus from a cryopreserved embryo. This fetus, like the child with Down syndrome in the present study, had developed from an embryo that was cryopreserved at the pronucleate stage. The possibility that there may be a link between the cryopreservation process and chromosomal abnormalities was not substantiated in a study comparing the transfer of cryopreserved embryos and fresh embryos[6]; there was no chromosomal abnormality reported in 283 infants conceived after transfer of cryopreserved embryos, but chromosomal abnormalities were observed in five of 961 infants after transfer of fresh embryos. The process of cryopreservation therefore may not increase the risk of chromosomal abnormalities in live-born infants, possibly because abnormal embryos are lost in the cryopreservation–thawing process, or early fetal losses occur because of abnormal chromosomes.

It has been previously reported that about 20–30% of embryos may not survive the cryopreservation–thawing process[26,27]. The reasons for this are not clearly understood but may be related to freezing[28].

Those embryos that survive the cryopreservation–thawing process may be a self-selected group in which the risk of a minor congenital anomaly or a major congenital anomaly is similar to the risk in normally conceived children. Animal experiments suggest that freezing does not appear to be mutagenic, and that background radiation of frozen embryos does not produce abnormal offspring[29]. A more detailed investigation in mice from cryopreserved embryos has suggested other effects at follow-up: on body weight, pre-weaning development, behavior and mandible morphometry[28]. Since some of these findings were in adult animals only, it is possible that the effects of embryo freezing and thawing may be delayed, therefore not yet detected.

Other studies

Children conceived from embryo cryopreservation are theoretically at risk of adverse outcomes, these risks being in addition to those experienced by those born from standard IVF. In addition, they are prone to risks well known to IVF pregnancies. These were summarized in Table 1.1. Very few follow-up studies have been performed on these children and all have inadequacies. The studies that have been performed are those that are obstetric oriented and those involving children beyond the perinatal period. Four papers, which report obstetric/perinatal studies in patients who conceived after replacement of cryopreserved embryos, are now discussed.

Frydman and co-workers[30] described the outcome of 50 pregnancies occurring over a 2-year period. One pregnancy was terminated at 22 weeks' gestation because of severe fetal malformations, one child was born prematurely and a high incidence of breech presentation at term in singleton pregnancies was noted. The study was largely descriptive.

Heijnsbroek and colleagues[31], in an observational study of pregnancy outcome of the first 30 women who conceived after transfer of cryopreserved and subsequently thawed embryos, gave brief information about the children. Infants were of above-average birth weight with no congenital anomalies.

In a more detailed study (referred to earlier in the chapter), the characteristics and perinatal outcome of babies conceived from cryopreserved embryos was performed by Wada and associates[6]. In this retrospective study of 232 consecutive births (which used equivalent IVF births for controls) there were similar mean gestational age, birth weight and perinatal mortality rates in the two groups. The paper claimed that major malformations in the cryopreserved group were significantly lower than in the IVF group. In this study no reference was made as to how congenital abnormalities were assessed, and by whom. Neither was there reference to how many births there were from pregnancies arising from these IVF and cryopreserved embryos. If these differed significantly, there may well have been a 'filtering effect' in the form of early spontaneous abortion or even earlier so-called 'chemical pregnancy' resulting in distortion of the apparent congenital abnormality rate (because of the tendency for pregnancies that are abnormal to abort spontaneously).

FIVNAT, the French IVF registry, examined files from 15 676 thawed embryo transfers[32], but could only relate the patient details to the original cycle giving rise to the frozen embryo in 8438 cycles. Abortion and ectopic pregnancies were noted to be similar to fresh transfers and multiple pregnancy, prematurity and low birth rate were noted to be lower than standard IVF, but only 53.4% of records were ascertained.

Wennerholm and co-workers[33] set out to evaluate the obstetric and neonatal outcomes in 270 infants (163 singleton, 98 twins and nine triplets.) Their conclusions after comparison of these children with two control groups (conventional IVF and normally conceived children) were similar to those of Sutcliffe *et al.*[34,35], that cryopreservation did not seem to influence fetal development adversely, and no increased perinatal risk was found.

There are only three studies specifically looking at these children beyond the postnatal period in the medical literature. The first study is the British study discussed above[34,35]. A more recent paper by Olivennes and colleagues[36], a study of 82 children aged 1–9 years old, confirmed the findings of Sutcliffe's group that these children were more likely to be born prematurely and from multiple births, but were of normal intelligence with a normal congenital malformation rate. This study did not use controls and did not make a detailed attempt to assess these children developmentally. Intellectual progress was inferred (probably correctly) by retrospective assessments of scholastic achievement in those children older than 5 years (i.e. school age.) The authors criticized the paper of Sutcliffe *et al.* by claiming that his study did not review the whole population concerned, however, we can confirm that more than 90% of eligible children were studied.

Finally Wennerholm and associates[37] assessed 255 children from cryopreserved embryos, matched for maternal age, parity, single or twin pregnancy and date of delivery with equal numbers (255) of fresh IVF and normally conceived children (252). In this study the main end-point was growth, with secondary end-points being chronic illness, major malformations, cumulative incidence of common diseases and 'development' during the first 18 months. This was a strong study for growth parameter outcome, but the developmental screening relied on records from child health centers, and the few relatively crude indices used would have detected only gross problems and made no allowance for interobserver error. Wennerholm and colleagues concluded that 'although the cryopreservation process did not adversely affect growth, minor handicaps, behavioural disturbances, learning difficulties, and dysfunction of attention/perception could not be ruled out at this age.' It seems likely that minor problems could not be detected using the study design/methods.

In common with other studies performed to examine outcome after various types of IVF, all the studies mentioned above are weak with respect to congenital anomaly rates. For confident assessment of birth defects let us consider conditions that normally affect 2% of births. To detect a doubling in that level of risk using a 5% one-tailed test of significance, and to ensure an 80% chance of detecting such an excess, we would need 1000 children from frozen embryos and 1000 control children. For a condition that normally affects 1/1000 births, the corresponding number of children would be 20 000 in each group.

CONCLUSION

Cryopreservation of human embryos may confer considerable benefits by increasing the number of pregnancies in an IVF program. However, couples who are planning pregnancy by assisted conception may wish to know about potential hazards and outcomes in children born after cryopreservation. The modest numbers of children available in the British study[34,35] was offset by the thorough examination of each child by one person.

This allowed an assessment, for the first time, of various minor congenital anomalies, which occur in a larger proportion of children than major congenital anomalies. Although there was an increased incidence of multiple pregnancies and of preterm births in the cryopreserved embryo group, none of the children had a major disability such as cerebral palsy. Children born after replacement of cryopreserved embryos appear to be healthy, but studies performed to date are few, and limited primarily by their size. The establishment of a birth registry involving at least one nation is the only way to achieve specific answers to the question of congenital abnormality rates.

REFERENCES

1. Trounson A, Mohr L. Human pregnancy following cryopreservation, thawing and transfer of an eight cell stage human embryo. *Nature (London)* 1983;305:707–9
2. Troup SA, Matson PL, Critchlow JD, *et al.* Cryopreservation of human embryos at the pronucleate, early cleavage, or expanded blastocyst stages. *Eur J Obstet Gynecol Reprod Biol* 1991;38:133–9
3. Cohen J, Simons RS, Fehilly CB, *et al.* Birth after replacement of hatching blastocyst cryopreserved at expanded blastocyst stage. *Lancet* 1985;8429:647
4. Lassalle B, Testart J, Renard J-P. Human embryo features that influence the success of cryopreservation with the use of 1,2 propanediol. *Fertil Steril* 1985;44:645–51
5. Whittingham DG. Principles of embryo cryopreservation. In Ashwood Smith MJ, Farrant J, eds. *Low Temperature Preservation in Medicine and Biology*. Tunbridge Wells: Pitman Medical, 1980;65–84
6. Wada I, Macnamee C, Wick K, *et al.* Birth characteristics and perinatal outcome of babies conceived from cryopreserved embryos. *Hum Reprod* 1994;9:543–6
7. Australian *in vitro* fertilisation collaborative group. High incidence of preterm births and early losses in pregnancy after *in vitro* fertilisation. *Br Med J (Clin Res Ed)* 1985;291:1160–3
8. MRC Working Party on Children Conceived by *In Vitro* Fertilisation. Births in Great Britain resulting from assisted conception, 1978–87. *Br Med J* 1990;300:1229–33
9. Tan SL, Doyle P, Campbell S, *et al.* Obstetric outcome of *in vitro* fertilisation pregnancies compared with normally conceived pregnancies. *Am J Obstet Gynecol* 1992;167:778–84
10. Freidman R, Forman R, Belaisch-Allart J, *et al.* An obstetric analysis of 50 consecutive pregnancies after transfer of cryopreserved embryos. *Am J Obstet Gynecol* 1989;160:209–13
11. Sutcliffe AG, DeSouza SW, Cadman J, *et al.* Outcome in children from cryopreserved embryos. *Arch Dis Child* 1995;72:290–3
12. Olsen J. The association between birth weight, placenta weight, pregnancy duration, subfecundity and child development. *Scand J Soc Med* 1994;22:213–18
13. Rossiter EJ. The Geelong study. *Acta Pediatr* 1993;82(suppl 392):1–55
14. Ounsted M, Scott A, Moar V. Delivery and development: to what extent can one associate cause and effect? *J R Soc Med* 1980;73:786–92
15. Rothenberg PB, Varga PE. The relationship between age of mother and child health and development. *Am J Pediatr Health* 1981;71:810–17
16. The Scottish low birth weight study: I. Survival, growth, neuromotor and sensory impairment. *Arch Dis Child* 1992;67:675–81

17. Marlow N, D'Souza SW, Chiswick ML. Neurodevelopmental outcome in babies weighing less than 2001 at birth. *Br Med J* 1987;294:1582–6
18. Yovich J, Barry T, French N, Grauaug A. Developmental assessments on twenty *in vitro* fertilisation (IVF) infants at their first birthday. *J In Vitro Fertil Embryo Transfer* 1986;3:253–7
19. Morin NC, Wirth H, Johnson DH, *et al.* Congenital malformations and psychosocial development in children conceived by *in vitro* fertilisation. *J Paediatr* 1989; 115:222–7
20. Brandes J, Scher A, Itskovits J, *et al.* Growth and development of children conceived by *in vitro* fertilisation. *Paediatrics* 1992;90:424–9
21. Huntley M. *The Griffiths Mental Development Scales. From Birth to 2 Years. Manual* (Revision). United Kingdom: Association for Research in Infant and Child Development
22. D'Souza SW, Rivlin E, Cadman J, *et al.* Children conceived by *in vitro* fertilisation after fresh embryo transfer. *Arch Dis Child* 1997;76:F70–4
23. Biggers JD. *In vitro* fertilization and embryo transfer in human beings. *N Engl J Med* 1981;304:336–42
24. Angell R, Aitken P, van Look P, *et al.* Chromosome abnormalities in human embryos after *in-vitro* fertilisation. *Nature (London)* 1983;303:336–7
25. Rizk B, Edwards RG, Nicolini U, *et al.* Edwards' syndrome after the replacement of cryopreserved–thawed embryos. *Fertil Steril* 1991;55:208–10
26. Sathanandan M, Macnamee MC, Rainsbury P, *et al.* Replacement of frozen–thawed embroyos in artificial and natural cycles: a prospective semi-randomised study. *Hum Reprod* 1991;6:685–7
27. Wada I, Matson PL, Troup SA, *et al.* Outcome of treatment subsequent to the elective cryopreservation of all embryos from women at risk of the ovarian hyperstimulation syndrome. *Hum Reprod* 1992;7:962–6
28. Duliost E. Long-term effects of embryo freezing in mice. *Proc Natl Acad Sci USA* 1995;92:589–93
29. Whittingham DG, Lyon MF, Glenister PH. Long-term storage of mouse embryos at −196 degrees C: the effect of background radiation. *Genet Res* 1977;29:171–81
30. Frydman R, Forman R, Belaisch-Allart J, *et al.* An obstetric analysis of 50 consecutive pregnancies after transfer of cryopreserved embryos. *Am J Obstet Gynecol* 1989; 160:209–13
31. Heijnsbroek I, Helmerorst FM, van den Berg-Helder AF, *et al.* Follow-up of 30 pregnancies after embryo cryopreservation. *Eur J Obstet Gynaecol Reprod Biol* 1995; 59:201–4
32. FIVNAT evaluation of frozen embryo transfers from 1987 to 1994 [in French]. *Contracept Fertil Sex* 1996;24:700–5
33. Wennerholm UB, Hamberger L, Nilsson L, *et al.* Obstetric and perinatal outcome of children conceived from cryopreserved embryos. *Hum Reprod* 1997;12:1819–25
34. Sutcliffe AG, D'Souza SW, Cadman J, *et al.* Outcome in children from cryopreserved embryos. *Arch Dis Child* 1995;72:290–3
35. Sutcliffe AG, D'Souza SW, Cadman J, *et al.* Minor congenital anomalies, major congenital malformations and development in children conceived from cryopreserved embryos. *Hum Reprod* 1995;10:3332–7
36. Olivennes F, Scheider Z, Remy V, *et al.* Perinatal outcome and follow-up of 82 children aged 1–9 years old conceived from cryopreserved embryos. *Hum Reprod* 1996;11:1565–8
37. Wennerholm UB. Postnatal growth and health in children born after cryopreservation as embryos. *Lancet* 1998;351:1085–90

4

Children born after intracytoplasmic sperm injection

'In completing one discovery we never fail to get an imperfect knowledge of others of which we could have no idea before, so that we cannot solve one doubt without creating several new ones'

Joseph Priestley, 1733–1804

In this chapter there is a comprehensive review of all that is known about children conceived by intracytoplasmic sperm injection (ICSI), with consideration of some aspects of the male infertility problems that were the stimulus for the development of ICSI. This description is in three parts: first concerning male infertility; second considering what extra risks there may be to ICSI-conceived children over and above IVF *per se*; and third a review and interpretation of all that is known about ICSI children to date.

ICSI AND MALE FACTOR INFERTILITY

ICSI was developed in Belgium by a pediatrician, Andre Van Steirteghem, and colleagues[1,2] following the relatively poor success rates arising from other *in vitro* fertilization (IVF) methods for male factor problems (Table 4.1). The technique of injecting spermatozoa into oocytes had been described prior to this, using hamster, rat and mouse eggs[3–5].

Male factor infertility contributes to approximately 40% of the problems of infertile couples[6,7]. Male factor infertility has a complex etiology beyond the scope of this book. However, Figure 4.1 summarizes the factors contributing to normal spermatogenesis. At the present time in the UK approximately one in 100 births follow IVF, 25–40% by the ICSI technique.

Table 4.1 Techniques for assisted fertilization using spermatozoa from severely subfertile men

Technique	*Year*	*Described by*
Zona splitting	1987	Laws-King *et al.*[89]
Subzonal sperm microinjection	1988	Ng *et al.*[90]
Pharmaceutical enhancement	1990	Yovich *et al.*[91]
of sperm function	1993	Yovich *et al.*[92]
Electroporation	1992	Palermo *et al.*[2]
Microassisted approaches	1993	Fishel *et al.*[29]
ICSI	1992	Van Steirteghem *et al.*[1]

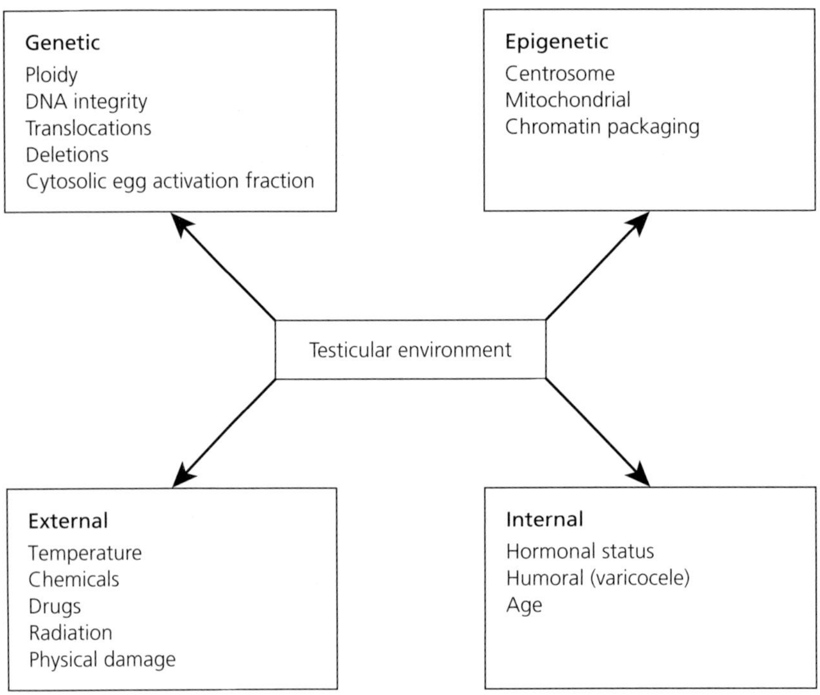

Figure 4.1 In order to assure healthy sperm and quality production there must be a proper testicular environment

In Belgium, ICSI is used in 60% of IVF procedures. Therefore, a minimum of one in 400 total births involve the ICSI procedure (in Western countries). Prior to the introduction of ICSI, men with oligozoospermia (a sperm count of < 5 000 000/ml), asthenozoospermia and teratozoospermia were unable to reproduce using conventional IVF techniques. ICSI has been rapidly introduced worldwide; more than 20 000 children had been born by 1997[8]. Unfortunately, because there was no animal model on which to test the technique (i.e. no infertile primate similar to man), it was not possible to test the safety of this technique prior to its introduction. The theoretical concerns already listed in Chapter 1 have not been fully addressed regarding the technique's safety. One notable absence from reports to date is an analysis of any relationship between sperm subtypes such as oligozoospermia and the developmental well-being of the children of these fathers. The development and congenital abnormalities in the children of males with various sperm subtypes are one aspect of the ongoing UK developmental outcome study of ICSI-conceived children. The data presented in this chapter drawn from this study have already been more fully published[9,10].

SOME THEORETICAL CONCERNS ABOUT THE USE OF ICSI

The subject of human infertility and the contribution made to it by genetic and chromosomal factors is complex. Penrose[11] suggested that infertile humans be considered in three categories with respect to these factors. In the first group he placed those individuals who carry a 'lethal condition' and who are infertile simply because they do not survive to reproductive age. Their genes kill them or chromosomal aberrations that they carry result in 'pregnancy wastage' exemplified by miscarriage, stillbirth and neonatal infant death. The chromosomally abnormal lethal and sublethal types in this group include most autosomal trisomies, triploidy and other unbalanced or aneuploid types.

In the second group, Penrose placed those individuals who are rendered infertile by hereditary mental or physical disorders that exclude them from establishing a normal heterosexual relationship. Individuals with such 'hereditary conditions' would include those with some of the sex chromosomal aneuploidies.

The third group with which this discussion is mainly concerned includes those individuals whose general health is not seriously disturbed by the abnormalities they carry, but who show infertility through some genetic or chromosomal condition that specifically affects the gonads. Members of this group, the 'infertile viable types', are likely to wish to reproduce, and their subsequent childlessness may lead them to seek advice at a clinic dealing with infertility. This has led to a number of cytogenetic investigations being carried out in such patients. Some theoretical concerns relevant to fathers needing ICSI are now discussed with a summary overview given in Tables 4.2 and 4.3.

Table 4.2 Intracytoplasmic sperm injection – independent problems

(1) Male gamete carrying genetic anomalies

- (a) cystic fibrosis mutations (epididymal spermatozoa from men with CBAVD)
- (b) Y-chromosome deletions
- (c) aneuploidy
- (d) ? lack of imprinting genes (when injecting spermatid nuclei)

(2) Male gamete with structural defects

- (a) lack of centrosome activity (when injecting spermatid nuclei)
- (b) deficit of cytoskeletal sperm proteins (calicin, actin, tubulin, centrin, etc). potentially responsible for round-headed sperm, severe forms of teratozoospermia and microtubule nucleation
- (c) lack of a particular isoform of creatine phosphokinase

(3) Anomalies of sperm activating 'factors' (signals for oocyte activation)
(4) Potential for incorporating sperm mitochondrial DNA
(5) Female gamete anomalies (oocyte aging-related)

CBAVD, congenital bilateral absence of the vas deferens

Table 4.3 Intracytoplasmic sperm injection – dependent problems (related to the technique itself)

(1) Injection of foreign, sperm-associated, plasmid DNA into the ooplasm and the risk of transgenic children or assimilation of infectious particles
(2) Injection of biochemical contaminants (from the medium)
(3) Mechanical oocyte activation (parthenogenesis)
(4) Physical and biochemical disturbance of the ooplasm
(5) Damage to the separating chromosomes in the second meiotic spindle
(6) Human in charge of sperm selection and site of injection

Morphology

Sperm of abnormal morphology, so-called teratozoospermia, are sometimes used in ICSI and these have an abnormal phenotype (e.g. malformed tails). There is no evidence in general that the phenotype of an individual spermatozoon reflects the genotype it carries (abnormal sperm phenotypes, such as teratozoospermia, have normal genotypes but are unlikely to fertilize an ovum). Rare examples of post-meiotic gene expression affecting sperm function, such as the T-locus in mice, are the exception rather than the rule[12]. Indeed, reflection on the evolution of fertilization, and the importance of random recombination of genotypes in Mendelian genetics, suggests that there are probably fundamental reasons why this is so[13].

In general the 'interests' of the whole organism are served (or have been served) best in evolution by genetic systems that suppress haploid gene expression in gametes, so that the recombination is truly random and not affected by the short-term 'interests' of the gametes[14]. Severely dysfunctional spermatozoa are usually the products of a severely dysfunctional reproductive tract that may in turn have its basis in a genetic anomaly[15].

Inheritance

Whilst couples who need ICSI to reproduce do not escape from the basic rule of biology, namely that our children inherit their genes from their parents, we are largely ignorant as to the etiology of male infertility. The condition of congenital bilateral absence of the vas deferens (CBAVD) is an obvious example of an indication for ICSI. It is now known that this condition is associated with the presence of mutations in the gene complex controlling cystic fibrosis (CF)[16]. Mutations in the CF trans-membrane regulator gene complex are highly significantly associated with reduced fertilization rates using epididymal spermatozoa in men with CBAVD[16]. It is clear from simple Mendelian genetics that the CF gene complex mutations will be present in half the embryos produced, so that half of the male babies born may, like their fathers, suffer from CBAVD or epididymal blockage. While screening for CF is possible in embryos[17] and first-trimester fetuses[18], this serves to multiply the technological intervention load and raises the additional ethical dilemma of selective abortion. It exposes the male child to potentially similar need for assisted reproduction technologies (ART) in adult life. The CF variants that have CBAVD as their sole phenotype are not specifically tested for in any CF screening programs.

Apart from clear-cut cases such as CF and CABVD, it is likely that, as understanding advances, other genetic causes of 'unexplained' male infertility will emerge. For example, Young syndrome is a poorly characterized combination of obstructive azoospermia and chronic respiratory problems. In such cases spermatogenesis, duct development and sperm ciliary function appear normal, but blockage occurs through the accumulation of inspissated epididymal secretions[19]. While this clinical picture has been considered to be distinct from CF proper, Hirsh and colleagues[20] recently demonstrated that two of seven infertile men with obstructive azoospermia were carriers of the δf508 CF mutation. This mutation is normally only found in 1 in 25 to 1 in 30 of the North European population, and the authors advocated that CF screening and genetic counselling should

Table 4.4 Mendelian conditions of which one feature is male infertility

Young syndrome
Pseudovaginal perineoscrotal hypospadias; ppsh
Pseudohermaphroditism, male, with gynecomastia
Androgen receptor; ar
Noonan syndrome 1; ns1
Male pseudohermaphroditism: deficiency of testicular 17,20-desmolase; tdd
Adrenal hyperplasia, congenital, due to 21-hydroxylase deficiency
Cystic fibrosis; cf
Kartagener syndrome
Reifenstein syndrome
Apolipoprotein b; apob
Vas deferens, congenital bilateral aplasia of; cbavd
Dystrophia myotonica; dmpk
Deleted in azoospermia-like; dazl
Cystic fibrosis transmembrane conductance regulator; cftr
Cytochrome p450, subfamily xix; cyp19
Dipeptidyl carboxypeptidase 1; dcp1
Spermatogenesis arrest
Ubiquitin-conjugating enzyme e2b; ube2b
Ataxia-telangiectasia; at
Gonadotropin releasing hormone 1; gnrh1
Follicle stimulating hormone, beta polypeptide; fshb
Deleted in azoospermia; daz
Heat-shock 70-kd protein 2; hspa2
Spinal muscular atrophy i; sma1
Hypomagnesemia, primary
Cyclic AMP response element modulator; crem
Blepharophimosis, epicanthus inversus and ptosis; bpes
Germinal cell aplasia
Follicle stimulating hormone receptor; fshr
UDP-*N*-acetylglucosamine pyrophosphorylase 1; uap1
Retinitis pigmentosa 3; rp3
Spinal and bulbar muscular atrophy, X-linked 1; smax1
Calmegin; clgn
Retinohepatoendocrinological syndrome
Cerebellar ataxia and hypogonadotropical hypogonadism
Fragile site 16q22; fra16a
Kenny–Caffey syndrome

Source: Online Mendelian Inheritance in Man (OMIM,14/04/1999)

be considered for men with Young syndrome. Moving to other genetic abnormalities, it is well established that infertile men show an approximately ten-fold increase in chromosomal anomalies as compared with normal controls[21,22]. A list of some of the conditions in which a syndromic diagnosis is associated with a low sperm count is shown in Table 4.4. Many of these fathers can be helped to conceive by ICSI.

An increased risk of chromosomal anomalies has been reported in spermatazoa of oligozoospermic men[23,24]. The incidence of karyotypic anomalies is inversely related to the number of spermatozoa in the ejaculate[25,26]. There is an argument for both azoospermic and oligospermic patients to be checked for disordered spermatogenesis before any ICSI treatment is carried out, to reduce the risk of transmission of aneuploidy to children. In a study of 1082 ICSI children, the sex chromosome aneuploidy rate was 0.8% compared to 0.2% in the general population[27]. There are undoubtedly a proportion of men who benefit from ICSI who have a genetic anomaly that is at least related to, and possibly causes, their fertility problems. Microdeletions in Yq have been the subject of much investigation. Such deletions may be passed on to the next male generation by ICSI and may give rise to fertility problems. However, of greater concern are unknown gene defects in humans that could potentially cause spermatogenesis problems and also have other serious health consequences. There are mouse models with such genes for which there are known human homologs with devastating pathologies such as familial colon cancer (mlh-1[28], MSH2[29]). The role of such genes in human idiopathic male infertility remains to be determined. A recent report[30] suggested a link between male infertility and trinucleotide repeat expansion in the androgen-receptor gene. With ICSI this mutation could be inherited, and should further elongation of the trinucleotide repeat occur in future generations, there is the potential for an increased risk of neurodegenerative disease including spinobulbar muscular atrophy or Kennedy's disease. In addition to conditions associated with infertility, ICSI patients may also have a higher risk of potentially heritable disorders unrelated to fertility[31].

Consideration of the mechanisms described above could lead to an increased risk of each of the following adverse health outcomes among the pregnancies and children produced by ICSI: miscarriage, stillbirth, congenital anomaly, serious or chronic disease of childhood, pediatric developmental problems or delay, cancer and death. Adverse outcomes may manifest at any age, but investigation must inevitably begin during the childhood of the ICSI children, and therefore we concentrate on such outcomes.

Genomic imprinting

The nature of genomic imprinting, in which certain genes transmitted through the male germ cell lineage differ in expression from those derived, through the female, by differential DNA methylation[32], is only just being elucidated. Although the imprinted genes derived from the male appear to be concerned with placental function, as exemplified by loss of the maternal genome in benign trophoblast disease (hydatidiform mole), it is not clear when imprinting is complete in sperm formation. Pregnancies have recently been achieved by use of round spermatid nuclear injection – ROSNI[33]. The clear links between sperm dysfunction and imperfect nuclear condensation give rise to concern about using immature gametes for ICSI, at least until there is better understanding of when genomic imprinting occurs. Other techniques can also be used to overcome azoospermia, such as elongated spermatid injection (ELSI) which uses immature germ lines. Azoospermia was not considered as a male sub-category in the present analysis of children because it is an extreme form of oligozoospermia (which was considered). No children in this study were born after these more invasive techniques. Any azoospermic males in the cohort were treated using ICSI. Oligo-asthenoteratozoospermia (OAT) is arguably the most severe form of male infertility treated with ICSI. Mercan and colleagues[34] investigated the outcome of clinical pregnancies following ICSI, specifically comparing 62 OAT patients with the 217 patients who underwent ICSI for other indications. The outcome was judged to be similar with no overall difference for OAT compared with the conventional IVF group regarding implantation, clinical pregnancy, delivery and miscarriage rate. Mercan and colleagues concluded that, although there were slightly reduced fertility rates in OAT patients, their chances of delivery and pregnancy loss were similar to those of other patients undergoing ICSI. This was rather surprising, in view of the work by Chandley[35], demonstrating that the incidence of chromosomal anomalies in patients with severe OAT was significantly increased to 2.2% in a non-selected group of males with subfertility when compared with the general male population (0.7% to > 1.0%[36]). Larger numbers of OAT/ICSI pregnancies may demonstrate an increased risk of problems. It has also been found that the incidence of these anomalies was positively correlated with the severity of spermatogenic impairment[37,38]. In the study of Yoshida and co-workers[38], 1007 males whose chief complaint was infertility were karyotyped; 62 patients (6.2%) had abnormal karyotypes – sex chromosome abnormalities in 38 patients (3.8%) and autosomal chromosome abnormalities in 24 (2.4%). Deletion of DNA sequences in specific parts of the Y-chromosome long arm[39,40] has been demonstrated in 10–15% of severely oligo- and azoospermic 46,XY individuals. This is discussed further below. Johannisson and associates[41] showed that Robertsonian translocations of chromosomes 13 and 14 resulted in oligoasthenoteratozoospermia. In a more recent study, comparison of fluorescent *in situ* hybridization (FISH) labelling of chromosomes 7, 11, 12, 18 and X and Y of spermatozoa from nine OAT patients in an IVF program with spermatozoa from nine fertile donors revealed significant differences of rates of abnormalities (1.45% vs. 19.6%).

Although it is well known that the incidence of chromosomal anomalies is higher in patients with severe male factor infertility and that there is a theoretical risk of transmission of these anomalies, most of the studies to date have shown no difference in pregnancy outcome after ICSI when compared with conventional IVF[42–46]. Govaerts and co-workers[47] reported a slightly higher incidence of fetal malformations following ICSI.

Conversely, in two recent studies, the major congenital malformation rate identified at birth was found to be lower after ICSI compared with that after standard IVF involving 578 children[48] and 210 children[49]. Palermo and colleagues[48] also reported no increased incidence of congenital abnormalities in patients with severe oligozoospermia or teratozoospermia.

Previous studies have shown that the three basic semen parameters (motility, morphology and count) apparently had significant impact on pregnancy outcome after ICSI[42,44,50]. However, Bourne and co-workers[42] found that the fertilization rate was significantly lower in patients with OAT.

Testicular aging

Testicular aging affects simultaneously the individual and his lineage. In the individual, changes because of age in vascular, endocrine, blood–testis barrier and Sertoli cells lead to a decrease in numbers of spermatozoa and an alteration in their form and motility. These changes lead to a gradual decrease of fertility[51].

The links between advanced paternal age and several genetic conditions in humans have been recognized for many years[51,52]. These include the diverse dominant conditions achondroplasia, myositis ossificans, Apert syndrome and the sex-linked recessive conditions, Duchenne muscular dystrophy, hemophilia A and bilateral retinoblastoma. There is a strong association between unexplained male infertility and accelerated testicular aging, as manifest in ischemic disorders, mitochondrial DNA deletions, disordered oxidative phosphorylation and loss of control over free radical production[15].

DNA breakage

Human semen is known to carry oxidized DNA products, and amounts may be increased in those individuals with an enhanced risk of oxidative damage, such as cigarette smokers[53]. In such cases dietary antioxidants such as ascorbate can reduce the seminal levels of oxidised DNA products and may also improve semen quality in some men[54]. Simple incubation of spermatozoa *in vitro* can also result in significant increases in DNA breakage, both in humans[55] and in laboratory animals[56]. In support of this, Jursicova and associates in 1999[57] found in a mouse model of azoospermia that the high rates of DNA fragmentation in round spermatids could be reduced by the introduction of antioxidants.

Breakage of DNA in turn can lead to chromosomal damage[58]. This can be accelerated by mutagenic agents such as ethyl methanesulfonate and potentiated by depletion of free-radical scavenging molecules such as glutathione[59]. These changes are consistent with the general view that most sperm-derived genetic damage to embryos occurs through chromosomal rearrangement[60]. While there do not appear to be any reports that have addressed this question directly, the potential amounts of oxidized DNA, and thus the risk that spermatozoa carry chromosomal breakages, are likely to be elevated in infertile men for several reasons.

(1) Spermatozoa in subfertile men are exposed to abnormal amounts of reactive oxygen species and altered amounts of scavenging enzymes that control them, such as superoxide dismutase[61,62]. These highly reactive molecules are well-known mutagens.

(2) In men with impaired spermatogenesis as well as epididymal lesions, it is likely that increased epididymal transit times will lead to aging of gametes *in vivo*[63]. Artificially aging spermatozoa in the male tract of rabbits is known to result in increased chromosomal anomalies in resulting embryos and in increased embryonic mortality[64].

(3) There are significant associations between male subfertility and imperfect spermiation and nuclear condensation. This can lead to poor DNA protection. Single-stranded or denatured DNA can be detected by acridine orange fluorescence microscopy[65].

(4) The failure to control amounts of transition metals in culture media used in IVF is likely to increase oxidative risk to DNA through catalysis of free-radical production[66]. Many of the clinics in that study used commercially prepared media, which contain copper or iron. This is hazardous, especially in cases dealing with spermatozoa that may already be rendered dysfunctional through the generation of excessive oxygen species or the impairment of scavenging systems.

Chromosomal aberrations

Chromosomal aberrations play a major part in male infertility. The sex chromosomes are especially involved in abnormalities. Karyotypes such as 47,XXY and 46,XX lead to an arrest in spermatogenesis. Translocations between the two sex chromosomes have the same result, no matter which arms are involved. In contrast, after translocations between gonosomes and autosomes, the influence on fertility ranges between normal fertility and azoospermy. This also applies to inversions and structural polymorphisms of the Y-chromosome as well as to the configurations 47,XXY and 45,XO/46,XY. The effects of autosomal aberrations on male fertility are difficult to estimate. They range between normal reproduction, a higher risk of abortion, more malformed children and a spermatogenetic breakdown. This is valid for the whole aberration type as well as for the specific abnormalities. The most important aberrations are the translocations, especially the reciprocal ones. During the past few years pericentric and paracentric inversions have received more attention, because of improved staining techniques. Other autosomal aberrations, such as trisomy, ring formation or duplication/deletion, are rarely found in sterility statistics. In most cases they are not compatible with life. A third complex of subfertility as a result of chromosomal aberrations are meiotic anomalies during gametogenesis. In spite of heterogeneous manifestations this can lead to a reduction of spermatogenesis.

Y-chromosome microdeletions

Male children of ICSI fathers who have these deletions would inherit the deletions and therefore need ICSI as adults in order to reproduce (see below for further comment). This examination would be indicated in certain subgroups of fathers needing ICSI. Although it is not believed that there is any association between Y-chromosome microdeletions and other phenotypic abnormalities, this is an unproven assumption.

Human Y-chromosome deletions in Yq11 associated with male infertility

Human Y-chromosomal rearrangements thought to interfere with male infertility were first identified in the karyotypes of human male metaphase chromosomes 22 years ago. Tiepolo and Zuffardi[67] observed terminal deletions of the long chromosome arm in six sterile men with azoospermia. It was consequently postulated that at least one genetic Y factor essential for male germ-cell development is located in distal Yq11, as these Y deletions seemed to result in 'azoospermia'. This Y factor was defined as azoospermia factor (AZF).

The general regions on the long arm of the Y chromosome relevant to infertility are found in deletion intervals 5 and 6[68]. The AZF candidate genes so far described are the YRRM[68] and DAZ (deleted in azoospermia)[69] gene families. Neither has been fully characterized. There have been numerous clinical studies in which DNA derived from the blood of azoospermic or severely oligozoospermic males has been screened using Y-linked sequence-tagged sites (STS)[68,70,71]. These studies demonstrate that the frequency of microdeletions in patients being treated with ICSI is in the range of 9–30% depending on patient selection criteria.

In a paper by Kent-First and associates[68] that investigated the incidence and possible relevance of Y-linked microdeletions in babies born after ICSI and their infertile fathers, it was suggested that it may be possible to predict the potential of inheriting Y-linked microdeletions, and likewise the ramifications of such inheritance. In a study by Stuppia and co-workers[72], a quarter of men with idiopathic oligoazoospermia were found to have microdeletions of different types in interval 6 of Yq11.

Perturbations of fertility-related genes are not life threatening and, as reproductive technologies such as ICSI improve, the chances for achieving a pregnancy will increase. It is likely that the DAZ and YRRM (RBM) gene families both have roles in the complicated process of spermatogenesis. However, microdeletions occurring in infertile patients between AZFb and AZFc suggest that other yet uncharacterized spermatogenesis-related genes or gene copies may exist.

Mutation events

Mutation events leading to Y-linked microdeletions may occur as pre- or post-meiotic *de novo* germ line mutations in a fertile male. If a son is produced he may inherit the microdeleted Y chromosome and exhibit infertility. Such an individual who does not possess an intact Y chromosome in his soma or in his germ cell lineage may resort to ICSI, and produce sons who also inherit the infertility-associated microdeletions. Mutation events leading to microdeletions may also occur as post-zygotic *de novo* events in the infertile propositus, although this individual will probably be mosaic for an intact Y and a Y with microdeletions.

CUMULATIVE EMPIRICAL EVIDENCE TO DATE AND ITS LIMITATIONS

Evidence of chromosomal anomalies in children conceived using ICSI was reviewed recently[73]. From 1082 prenatal tests in an unselected group of ICSI pregnancies it was revealed that 28 (2.6%) were abnormal, ten were inherited chromosomal anomalies and 18 *de novo* (nine sex chromosomal and nine autosomal). The father was the carrier in all but one case of the inherited anomalies. There was an increased risk of both *de novo* sex chromosomal anomalies (four-fold expected) and *de novo* autosomal anomalies (excluding trisomy 21, structural chromosomal anomalies five-fold expected).

Major congenital anomalies have been investigated by a number of groups. One of the initial series was concerned with 423 ICSI children[46] and the data were subjected to a detailed independent review[74]. The original investigators concluded that there was no evidence of an excess of major birth defects, whereas the independent reviewers concluded that there was a two-fold excess. The latter work, however, was fundamentally flawed. It contradicted one of the basic rules of population studies in that it failed to compare like populations. The Western Australian birth registry gets its data from an indigent population that includes, for example, a proportion of aboriginal native Australians. This ethnic group, like any other, has a predisposition to certain congenital abnormalities. The notion that norms from their group can be meaningfully compared to those from Belgium is deluded. Apples and oranges are both fruit, but one is citrus, one not so! Mitchell[75] in an accompanying editorial suggested that this discrepancy arose as a result of different definitions and methods of ascertainment of birth defects. Mitchell also discussed apparent differences between the expansion of the original 423 ICSI children to 877[76] and a further series of 578 ICSI children conceived in New York, and concluded that different methods of ascertainment of birth defects could explain a large element of the apparent discrepancy in the risk estimates. Mitchell concluded that the data overall suggested that ICSI children do not experience a substantially increased risk of all major birth defects considered together. However, he also noted that the number of ICSI children available for analysis at the time were insufficient to rule out moderate increases in the risk of all major birth defects or substantial increases in the risk of specific defects.

Since the Mitchell report there have been reports from Denmark based on 730 ICSI children[77] and from Sweden based on 1139 ICSI children[78]. The Swedish study reported that the risk of hypospadias among the ICSI children was three-fold that expected from the general population. Each of these studies emphasized the need for a sufficiently large study with an appropriate control group for satisfactorily addressing the question of the risk of congenital anomalies among ICSI children.

OTHER CONCERNS

In theory, as mentioned in previous chapters, there are other potential concerns about children conceived after ICSI. Although the main concerns are regarding their fathers' genetic background, those regarding the physical process of ICSI also require discussion.

Chemical toxicity

Exposure of sperm to different potential chemical toxins is referred to above and is not discussed further. Such exposure is not specific to ICSI and one would expect evidence from conventional IVF if there were harmful effects from these 'toxins'. However, to prevent the sperm tail damaging the egg, paralyzing chemicals are used that are not used in other forms of IVF.

Mechanical effects

More important are the mechanical aspects of ICSI (Figure 4.2). First the entire sperm, not only the sperm nucleus, enters the ovum. Compounding this in ICSI, one sperm is selected by the embryologist to be injected, whereas in a normal ejaculate there are over 20 000 000 sperm in competition. Although the embryologist selects a morphologically 'normal' sperm this is clearly not the same as the competitive selection, which occurs in natural conception and to a degree in other forms of ART.

Furthermore, the embryologist orientates the injection supposedly to avoid the risk of physical trauma to the invisible first meiotic spindle. However, it has recently been shown that this supposed orientation, which relies on the position of the visible polar body, is fundamentally flawed. In an elegant series of experiments by Hewitson and colleagues[79] it has been shown that in natural fertilization the sperm head enters the egg from any direction (apparently randomly). Furthermore, the relationship of the first meiotic spindle to the first polar body is not fixed. Therefore, the orientation (3 o'clock or 9 o'clock) of the injection micropipette based on a supposed fixed relationship between the visible polar body and the invisible first meiotic spindle is based on unjustified assumptions. This lends further support to concern that ICSI may be causing unknown damage to the egg

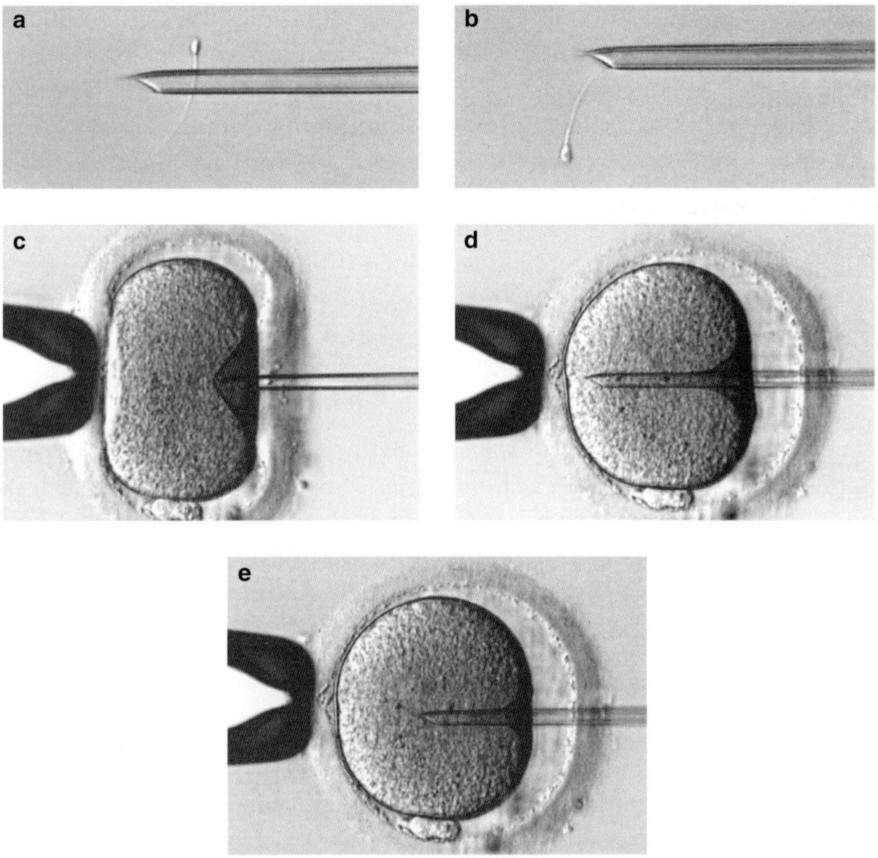

Figure 4.2 Intracytoplasmic sperm injection techniques. (a) The spermatozoon is immobilized, and then (b) aspirated into the injection pipette. (c) The zona pellucida is transversed. (d) The injection pipette is plunged deeply into the ooplasm in an effort to pierce the oolemma. (e) The spermatozoon is deposited and the injection pipette is gently withdrawn. Figures reproduced by kind permission of Lucinda L. Veeck, MLT, hDSC, Cornell University Medical College, New York, USA

during fertilization. The calcium fluxes and membrane potential changes following ICSI are different from those after normal sperm–oocyte fusion[80]. Early embryonic development is a complex cascade of critically timed molecular events. This cascade is finely controlled by genetic signals, which are not yet fully understood. Hence, manipulation at the level of sperm–egg interaction to this extent (e.g. spermatozoon oocyte injection) may disrupt many critical molecular events downstream. Aytoz and co-workers[81] examined 1427 pregnancies following ICSI and found amongst pregnancies in which more severely affected sperm was used that the rate of intrauterine death was higher than in less severely affected sperm. Sperm quality was judged according to concentration < 5 million; progressive motility < 20% and normal morphology approximately 20%, and was graded according to the presence of these criteria.

This could possibly affect embryonic or fetal developmental problems. Luetjens and colleagues[82] commented on non-random chromosome positioning in human sperm and proposed that this may lead to a higher rate of sex chromosome anomalies. These authers observed that, whereas in ICSI the apical tip of the sperm nucleus adjacent to the perinuclear theca remains condensed for longer than the basal part of the nucleus, these structures are lost uniformly at the egg cortex in natural/conventional IVF conceptions. The authors proposed that this may lead to mitotic errors in the distribution of the X-chromosome during first cleavage; such a positioning of the sex chromosome could lead to an increase of sex chromosomal anomalies following ICSI.

SUMMARY OF POTENTIAL PROBLEMS WITH ICSI

A summary of problems associated with ICSI was listed in Tables 4.2 and 4.3. These relate to the technique itself and to those independent of the technique.

SUMMARY FINDINGS FROM THE STUDY OF ICSI CHILDREN

The UK population

Tables 4.5 and 4.6 have been chosen from my ICSI study to highlight certain issues concerning ICSI-conceived children. The study was performed by me and involved 208 ICSI-conceived children with 221 naturally conceived 'control' children. The study of these children is ongoing and is currently an assessment at 5 years in collaboration with Belgian, Greek, Danish and Swedish investigators.

From the tables it can be seen that a variety of sperm sub-categories have been considered for outcome: oligozoospermia, teratozoospermia, asthenozoospermia (as defined above), a combined category of oligoasthenteratzoospermia, motility categories and morphology categories. Motility was considered via categories other than asthenozoospermia. The reason for this was partially pragmatic; the available male factor data lend

Table 4.5 Neurodevelopmental outcomes of case children according to male sperm analysis. Standard deviations are shown in parentheses

		Mean Griffiths Score	
Sperm abnormality	*No. of cases*	*Cases*	*Controls*
Motility			
< 30%	92	98.22 (9.48)	
30–59%	70	98.08 (12.85)	
> 60%	46	97.78 (10.71)	
Morphology			
normal	112	99.66 (10.67)	
abnormal	96	96.21 (11)	
Oligoasthenoteratozoospermia			
yes	32	100.25 (7.55)	
no	176	96.78 (11.41)	
Oligozoospermia*			
yes	98	98.09 (10.98)	98.69 (9.99)
no	110	96.68 (12.61)	
Asthenozoospermia			
yes	74	98.49 (11.26)	
no	134	96.47 (12.72)	
Teratozoospermia+			
yes	65	98.92 (8.73)	
no	100	96.61 (13.17)	
Sperm count < 5 x 10^6			
yes	87	98.81 (10.98)	
no	121	96.47 (12.72)	

*In this case, less than 20 x 10^6; +available data

to analysis in categories of < 30%, 30–59% and 60% or more. This also allowed examination for trends.

Some men, who had fathered children in a previous relationship without the use of artificial reproductive techniques, had subsequently had a vasectomy, so becoming infertile. Their semen should not be at risk of passing on putative genetic problems to their children. Likewise, unfortunate men who had naturally conceived children prior to chemotherapy and then later required ICSI should not be at risk, because their sperm was stored prior to treatment. These two groups were considered together in the analysis as an internal control group and are referred to as the 'previous pregnancy group'. It could, however, be argued that these two groups should have been considered individually, because freezing sperm after chemotherapy may have had deleterious effects on the sperm or

Table 4.6 Griffiths scales of mental development. Mean scores with SD in parentheses

	Study children (n = 208)		*Control children* (n = 221)	
	Mean	*95% CI*	*Mean*	*95% CI*
Chronological age (months)*	17.23 (3.33)	16.78–17.68	18.04 (3.06)	17.63–18.45
Griffiths quotient	98.08 (10.93)	96.59–99.57	98.69 (9.99)	97.38–100.00
Mental age (months)*	16.90 (3.77)	16.39–17.41	17.73 (3.29)	17.30–18.16
Sub-quotients				
locomotor	93.1 (16.05)	90.92–95.28	95.39 (14.34)	93.5–97.27
personal/social	95.14 (15.41)	93.05–97.23	96.06 (15.29)	94.04–98.08
hearing and speech	106.47 (14.40)	104.51–108.43	105.15 (14.16)	103.29–107.01
eye–hand co-ordination	98.92 (14.73)	96.92–100.92	100.41 (14.21)	98.52–102.29
performance	96.31 (13.16)	94.51–98.11	96.29 (14.67)	94.34–98.23

*$p = < 0.05$

alternatively destroyed the 'weaker' sperm and thus have ameliorative effects, but numbers did not justify this analysis. This previous pregnancy group was able to fulfil two roles. First, they would be the group whose children *if* abnormal, and *if* compared with a normally conceived control group would be most likely to implicate the ICSI technique as damaging. In addition, they would form a control group for an internal comparison of ICSI-conceived children. If ICSI was to be implicated as harmful *per se*, the previous pregnancy group might show developmental delay or higher rates of congenital abnormalities. Family enquiry was made in all ICSI-conceived children with previous naturally conceived siblings regarding congenital abnormalities in those siblings. There were none identified.

Findings

It can be seen from Table 4.5 that children conceived from fathers with a variety of categories of sperm abnormality had reassuringly normal developmental outcome at a mean age of 18 months. It can be seen from Table 4.6 that overall congenital abnormality rates in children from fathers who had various sperm abnormalities were generally not significantly different from the control group. There is an important exception in that the children born to fathers who had oligozoospermia were more likely to have congenital abnormalities in relation to other sperm sub-categories combined. In addition, this group was more likely to have congenital abnormalities when compared with a subgroup of children whose fathers had conceived children naturally prior to ICSI. These results are reassuring with the exception of children born to oligozoospermic males. Later inclusion of a group of children conceived after ICSI treatment in Melbourne, Australia (seen by my colleague Dr Kerryn Saunders) provided reassurance that this apparent finding was a feature of the small group size for this kind of outcome. The main outcome of the UK study is shown in Table 4.5.

A review of other outcome studies of children born after ICSI

Despite theoretical concerns regarding children conceived after ICSI, little effort has been made to follow up these children. Studies of neurodevelopmental outcome have been restricted to those by Bonduelle and colleagues[27,83,84] and those by Bowen and colleagues[85]. All of these studies had design problems possibly leading to erroneous conclusions. Their findings were contradictory, with Bonduelle and colleagues finding normal development at age 2 years when ICSI children were compared to an

Table 4.7 Summary of what is known about congenital anomalies after ICSI (papers with smaller numbers not included)

Authors	*Number of ICSI-conceived children*	*Type and number of controls*	*Country of origin*	*Overall congenital anomaly rate; ICSI/control*
Wennerholm *et al.*[78]	1139	birth registry of Sweden, i.e. not controls specifically for the study	Sweden	risk of 1.75 × the average for Sweden of an anomaly (in reality a small background risk)
Bonduelle *et al.*[76]	877 (from 904 pregnancies)	none	Belgium	2.6% (normal) but suggestion of increased sex chromosome anomalies
Bonduelle *et al.*[87]	2889	2995 IVF-conceived children	Belgium	3.38% in ICSI vs. 3.79% in IVF
Ludwig[88]	3215	2807 naturally conceived controls	Germany	
Hansen *et al.*[93]	301	4000	Australia	8.6% in ICSI vs. 4.2% in naturally-conceived

IVF-conceived control group, whereas Bowen and colleagues found that ICSI-conceived 1-year-olds were more likely than an IVF or normally conceived control group to show moderate developmental delay. These studies are discussed in more detail in Chapter 1, and the study by Bowen and colleagues[85] was also the subject of a critique by Sutcliffe and co-workers[86]. At 5 years of age, the original cohort seen at 1 year by Bowen and co-workers seemed normal, as assessed by the Weschler Infant Intelligence Scales (WIPSI-R), thus contradicting their earlier findings.

Studies of outcome specifically to look at congenital anomalies include those by Bonduelle, Wennerholm and Ludwig. The most contemporary reports by Bonduelle's group[87] and Ludwig[88] were both presented at the *17th Annual Meeting of the European Society of Human Reproduction*, in July 2001. These are summarized in Table 4.7, along with those previously published by Wennerholm and colleagues[78]. None of these studies are robust enough to answer the question on the minds of all families and fertility clinics who have used ICSI: namely, is there a higher risk of birth defects

Table 4.8 Numbers of ICSI-conceived and control offspring required to detect a specified relative risk of a congenital anomaly

	Statistical power	
Relative risk	*80%*	*90%*
2	20 000	27 000
3	7000	9000
4	4000	5000

from ICSI? Ultimately, Bonduelle's group may address this issue with rising numbers of children seen at birth. Wennerholm's work is weak because of the small numbers of children involved, reflecting the small population of Sweden for this kind of study. The German study relied on a comparison between prospectively collected data on ICSI-conceived children and a single region's birth registry data. Mainz may reflect the population of the former West Germany but not the East German areas from where children were partially recruited. There is a higher environmental risk to children born in the eastern parts of Germany.

To put limitations on the present studies on ICSI-conceived children and congenital anomalies, consider the generality of major congenital anomalies, for which the birth prevalence is about 2% in the general population. If one wished to detect a two-fold increase in risk among ICSI children using a 5% one-tailed test of significance, then to guarantee an 80% (or 90%) chance of detecting this, one would require 1000 (or 1350) children in each of the ICSI and control groups. In practice it is unlikely that the risk of a spectrum of different serious congenital anomalies would be adversely affected by the ICSI procedure. Instead, experience indicates that, if there were to be an effect then it would affect specific types of congenital anomaly. Specific types of congenital anomaly rarely occur in the general population with a birth prevalence of more than one in 1000 births. For example, Down syndrome, anencephaly, spina bifida aperta, hydrocephaly and cleft lip (with or without cleft palate) all have a birth prevalence in the region of one in 1000 births. Consider a condition that affects one in 1000 births in the general population. If one intended to use a 5% one-tailed test of significance of the null hypothesis that the proportion of ICSI and control offspring affected are identical, then the numbers shown in Table 4.8 of ICSI (and an identical number of control) offspring would be required to achieve a specified statistical power to detect a specified

Table 4.9 Statistical power (%) to detect a specified standardized incidence ratio with a specified number of ICSI children

Standardized incidence ratio	Number of ICSI children 4000	5000	10 000	12 000	20 000
2	39	41	73	81	92
3	80	84	99	100	100
4	95	98	100	100	100

relative risk (Hawkins and colleagues, 2001, in an unpublished grant application called National ICSI Study, of which I am a member of the steering committee).

Childhood cancer

Another adverse health outcome for which the risk might be increased among the ICSI offspring is cancer. The risk of any cancer at any age could potentially be increased. However, the risk of childhood cancer among the ICSI offspring will not become apparent initially and therefore we need to consider the chance that studies of different sizes have of detecting an excess risk. The risk of a child in the general population developing any type of childhood cancer by the age of 5 years is about eight in 10 000. If one intended to use a 5% one-tailed test of significance of the null hypothesis that the risks are identical in the ICSI and general populations then the statistical power in Table 4.9 is achievable to detect a specified standardized incidence ratio with a specified number of ICSI offspring.

To summarize the maths

A prospective comparative cohort study that obtained consent from 5800 ICSI families producing singleton live births (assuming 70% of control families participated – which would provide about 4000 matched pairs of children for data collection and analysis) would provide about an 80% chance of detecting a four-fold increase in the risk of congenital anomalies that occur with a birth prevalence of one in 1000 in the general population. Such a study should be considered an absolute minimum to provide a useful international contribution to the outstanding issues relating to the adverse health risks associated with ICSI. A retrospective registry study involving 19 000 ICSI offspring would provide about a 90% chance of detecting a doubling in the risk of childhood cancer by 5 years of age.

This puts the achievements of researchers in the field (see Table 4.8) in a robust statistical perspective. It shows what might be the difficulties of performing such a study. The study that we are proposing in the UK will cost £1 600 000 and take 3 years to perform. It would be impossible to perform this study in the USA, because of lack of co-operation from some clinics, and it would also be impossible within a meaningful time frame to consider trying to answer this question in a country such as Sweden with a low population.

Conclusions about what is known about ICSI-conceived children

It appears on the basis of available evidence to date that ICSI-conceived children do not differ in any major way from other IVF-conceived children. This is perhaps slightly surprising considering the extra theoretical risks to which their mode of conception is exposed. The ultimate question, which will be asked, of these children will be with regards to their own fertility. When counselling families about the risks, apart from referring in general terms to the above, one can specify what is certain. That is that a small proportion of ICSI-conceived male children will inherit from their fathers the same Y-chromosome deletion that they had. Nothing else can be said with certainty. The balance of evidence to date is that these children are healthy.

REFERENCES

1. Van Steirteghem AC, Nagy A, Liu J, *et al*. Intracytoplasmic sperm injection. *Assist Reprod Rev* 1993;3:160–3
2. Palermo G, Joris H, Devroey P, Van Steirteghem AC. Pregnancies after intracytoplasmic injection of single spermatozoon into an oocyte. *Lancet* 1992;340:17–18
3. Thadani VM. A study of hetero-specific sperm–egg interactions in the rat, mouse and deer mouse using *in vitro* fertilization and sperm injection. *J Exp Zool* 1980; 212:435–53
4. Makert CL. Fertilization of mammalian eggs by sperm injection. *J Exp Zool* 1983; 228:195–201
5. Uehara T, Yanagimachi R. Microsurgical injection of spermatozoa into hamster eggs with subsequent transformation of sperm nuclei into male pronuclei. *Biol Reprod* 1976;15:467–70
6. Hargreave TB. Introduction. In Hargreave TB, Soon TE, eds. *The Management of Male Infertility*. Singapore: PG Publishing
7. Skakkebaek NE, Giwercman A, de Kretser D. Pathogenesis and management of male infertility. *Lancet* 1994;343:1473–9
8. De Mouzon J, Lancaster P. World collaborative report on *in vitro* fertilization: preliminary data for 1995. *J Assist Reprod Hum Genet* 1997;14:251S–255S

9. Sutcliffe AG, Taylor B, Li J, *et al.* Children born after intracytoplasmic sperm injection: population control study. *Br Med J* 1999;318:704–5
10. Sutcliffe AG, Taylor B, Saunders K, *et al.* Outcome in the second year of life after *in-vitro* fertilisation by intracytoplasmic sperm injection: a UK case–control study. *Lancet* 2001:357:2080–4
11. Penrose LS. Genetical aspects of human infertility. *Proc R Soc London* 1933;159: 93–106
12. Hurst LD. A model for the mechanism of transmission ratio distortion and for *t*-associated hybrid sterility. *Proc R Soc London* 1993;253:83–91
13. Cummins JM. Evolution of sperm form: levels of control and competition. In Bavister BD, Cummins JM, Roldan ERS, eds. *Fertilization in Mammals*. Norwell, MA: Serono Symposia, 1990:51–64
14. Hurst LD. Selfish genes and meiotic drive. *Nature (London)* 1998;391:223
15. Cummins JM, Jequier AM. Treating male infertility needs more clinical andrology not less. *Hum Reprod* 1994;9:1214–19
16. Patrizio P, Asch RH, Handelin B, Silber SJ. Aetiology of congenital absence of vas deferens; genetic study of three generations. *Hum Reprod* 1993;8:215–20
17. Liu J, Lissens W, Devroey P, *et al.* Polymerase chain reaction analysis of the cystic fibrosis mutation in human blastomeres following oocyte injection of a single sperm from a carrier. *Prenat Diagn* 1993;13:873–80
18. McIntosh I, Lorenzo ML, Brock DJ. Frequency of delta F508 mutation on cystic fibrosis chromosomes in UK. *Lancet* 1989;2:1404–5
19. Handelsman DJ, Conway AJ, Boylan LM, Turtle JR. Young's syndrome: obstructive azoospermia and chronic sino-pulmonary infections. *N Engl J Med* 1984;310:3–9
20. Hirsh A, Williams C, Williamson B. Young's syndrome and cystic fibrosis mutation delta F508. *Lancet* 1993;342:118
21. Chandley AC. The chromosomal basis of human subfertility. *Br Med Bull* 1979;35; 181–6
22. Dutrillaux B, Rotman J, Gueguen J. Chromosomal factors in male infertility. In De Vere White R, ed. *Aspects of Male Infertility*. Baltimore, MD: Williams and Wilkins, 1982;89–102
23. Bernardini L, Martini E, Geraedts JP, *et al.* Comparison of gonosomal aneuploidy in spermatozoa of normal fertile men and those with severe male factor detected by *in-situ* hybridization. *Mol Hum Reprod* 1997;3:431–8
24. McInnes B, Rademaker A, Greene CA, *et al.* Abnormalities for chromosomes 13 and 21 detected in spermatozoa from infertile men. *Hum Reprod* 1998;13:2787–90
25. Yoshida A, Miura K, Shirai M. Cytogenetic survey of 1007 infertile males. *Urol Int* 1997;58:166–76
26. Van Assche E, Bonduelle M, Tournaye H, *et al.* Cytogenetics of infertile men. *Hum Reprod* 1996;11(suppl 4):1–24; discussion 25–6
27. Bonduelle M, Camus M, De Vos A, *et al.* Seven years of intracytoplasmic sperm injection and follow-up of 1987 subsequent children. *Hum Reprod* 1999;14(suppl 1): 243–64
28. Bronner CE, Baker SM, Morrison PT, *et al.* Mutation in the DNA mismatch repair gene homologue hMLH1 is associated with hereditary non-polyposis colon cancer. *Nature (London)* 1994;368:258–61
29. Fishel S, Dowell K, Timson J, *et al.* Micro-assisted fertilization with human gametes. *Hum Reprod* 1993;8:1780–4
30. Dowsing AT, Yong EL, Clark M, *et al.* Linkage between male infertility and trinucleotide repeat expansion in the androgen-receptor gene. *Lancet* 1999;354:640–3

31. Meschede D, Lemcke B, Behre HM, *et al.* Non-reproductive heritable disorders in infertile couples and their first degree relatives. *Hum Reprod* 2000;15:1609–12
32. Surani M, Sasaki H, Ferguson S, *et al.* The inheritance of germline specific epigenetic modifications during development. *Philos Trans R Soc London* 1993;339: 165–72
33. Silber SJ, Johnson L. Are spermatid injections of any clinical value? ROSNI and ROSI revisited. Round spermatid nucleus injection and round spermatid injection. *Hum Reprod* 1998;13:509–15
34. Mercan R, Lanzendorf SE, Mayer J Jr, *et al.* The outcome of clinical pregnancies following intracytoplasmic sperm injection is not affected by semen quality. *Andrologia* 1998;30:91–5
35. Chandley AC. The chromosomal basis of human subfertility. *Br Med Bull* 1979; 35;181–6
36. Lange R, Engel W. Chromosomal aberrations as a cause of male infertility. *Fertilitat* 1991;3:79–92
37. Retief AE, Van Zyl JA, Menkveld R, *et al.* Chromosome studies in 496 infertile males with a sperm count below 10 million/ml. *Hum Genet* 1984;66:162–4
38. Yoshida A, Miura K, Shirai M. Cytogenetic survey of 1007 infertile males. *Urol Int* 1997;58:166–76
39. Ma K, Inglis JD, Sharkey A, *et al.* A Y chromosome gene family with RNA-binding protein homology: candidates for the azoospermia factor AZF controlling human spermatogenesis. *Cell* 1993;75:1287–95
40. Kobayashi K, Mizuno K, Hida A, *et al.* PCR analysis of the Y chromosome long arm in azoospermic patients: evidence for a second locus required for spermatogenesis. *Hum Mol Genet* 1994;3:1965–7
41. Johannisson R, Schwinger E, Wolff HH, *et al.* The effect of 13;14 Robertsonian translocations on germ-cell differentiation in infertile males. *Cytogenet Cell Genet* 1993;63:151–5
42. Bourne H, Watkins W, Speirs A, Baker HW. Pregnancies after intracytoplasmic injection of sperm collected by fine needle biopsy of the testis. *Fertil Steril* 1995;64: 433–6
43. Mansour RT, Aboulghar MA, Serour GI, *et al.* The effect of sperm parameters on the outcome of intracytoplasmic sperm injection. *Fertil Steril* 1995;64:982–6
44. Oehninger S, Veeck L, Lanzendorf S, *et al.* Intracytoplasmic sperm injection: achievement of high pregnancy rates in couples with severe male factor infertility is dependent primarily upon female and not male factors. *Fertil Steril* 1995;64: 977–81
45. Sherins RJ, Thorsell LP, Dorfmann A, *et al.* Intracytoplasmic sperm injection facilitates fertilization even in the most severe forms of male infertility: pregnancy outcome correlates with maternal age and number of eggs available. *Fertil Steril* 1995; 64:369–75
46. Bonduelle M, Legein J, Buysse A, *et al.* Prospective follow-up study of 423 children born after intracytoplasmic sperm injection. *Hum Reprod* 1996;11: 1558–64
47. Govaerts I, Koenig I, Van den Bergh M, *et al.* Is intracytoplasmic sperm injection (ICSI) a safe procedure? What do we learn from early pregnancy data about ICSI? *Hum Reprod* 1996;11:440–3
48. Palermo G, Colombero L, Schattman G, *et al.* Evolution of pregnancies and initial follow-up of newborns delivered after intracytoplasmic sperm injection. *J Am Med Assoc* 1996;276:1893–7

49. Wennerholm UB, Bergh C, Hamberger L, *et al.* Obstetric and perinatal outcome of pregnancies following intracytoplasmic sperm injection. *Hum Reprod* 1996;11: 1113–9
50. Mansour RT, Aboulghar MA, Serour GI, *et al.* The effect of sperm parameters on the outcome of intracytoplasmic sperm injection. *Fertil Steril* 1995;64:982–6
51. Auroux M. La qualité du conceptus en fonction de l'age du père. *J Urol (Paris)* 1993;99;29–34
52. Lints F. *Genetics and Aging*, 1st edn. Basel: Karger, 1978
53. Fraga C, Motchnik P, Shigenaga M, *et al.* Ascorbic acid protects against endogenous oxidative DNA damage in human sperm. *Proc Natl Acad Sci USA*, 1991;88;11003–6
54. Dawson EB, Harris WA, Teter MC, Powell LC. Effect of ascorbic acid supplementation on the sperm quality of smokers. *Fertil Steril* 1992;58:1034–9
55. Martin RH, Rademaker AW, Ko E, *et al.* A comparison of the frequency and type of chromosomal abnormalities in human sperm after different sperm capacitation conditions. *Biol Reprod* 1992;47:268–70
56. Estop AM, Munne S, Jost LK, Evenson DP. Studies on sperm chromatin structure alterations and cytogenetic damage of mouse sperm following *in vitro* incubation. Studies on *in vitro*-incubated mouse sperm. *J Androl* 1993;14:282–8
57. Jurisicova A, Lopes S, Meriano J, *et al.* DNA damage in round spermatids of mice with a targeted disruption of the Pp1cgamma gene and in testicular biopsies of patients with non-obstructive azoospermia. *Mol Hum Reprod* 1999;5:323–30
58. Marder BA, Morgan WF. Delayed chromosomal instability induced by DNA damage. *Mol Cell Biol* 1993;13:6667–77
59. Evenson DP, Jost LK, Gandy J. Glutathione depletion potentiates ethyl methanesulfonate-induced damage to sperm chromatin structure. *Reprod Toxicol* 1993;7:297–304
60. Plachot M. Cytogenetic analysis of oocytes and embryos. *Ann Acad Med Singapore* 1992;21:538–44
61. Aitken RJ, Irvine DS, Wu FC. Prospective analysis of sperm–oocyte fusion and reactive oxygen species generation as criteria for the diagnosis of infertility. *Am J Obstet Gynecol* 1991;164:542–51
62. Kobayashi T, Miyazaki T, Natori M, Nozawa S. Protective role of superoxide dismutase in human sperm motility: superoxide dismutase activity and lipid peroxide in human seminal plasma and spermatozoa. *Hum Reprod* 1991;6:987–91
63. Johnson L. Evaluation of the human testis and its age-related dysfunction. *Prog Clin Biol Res* 1989;302:35–60; discussion 61–7
64. Tesh JM, Glover TD. Ageing of rabbit spermatozoa in the male tract and its effect on fertility. *J Reprod Fertil* 1969;20:287–97
65. Kosower NS, Katayose H, Yanagimachi R. Thiol-disulfide status and acridine orange fluorescence of mammalian sperm nuclei. *J Androl* 1992;13:342–8
66. Miesel R, Drzejczak PJ, Kurpisz M. Oxidative stress during the interaction of gametes. *Biol Reprod* 1993;49:918–23
67. Tiepolo L, Zuffardi O. Localization of factors controlling spermatogenesis in the nonfluorescent portion of the human Y chromosome long arm. *Hum Genet* 1976; 34:119–24
68. Kent-First MG, Kol S, Muallem A, *et al.* The incidence and possible relevance of Y-linked microdeletions in babies born after intracytoplasmic sperm injection and their infertile fathers. *Mol Hum Reprod* 1996;2:943–50
69. Reijo R, Lee TY, Salo P, *et al.* Diverse spermatogenic defects in humans caused by Y chromosome deletions encompassing a novel RNA-binding protein gene. *Nature Genet* 1995;10:383–93

70. Qureshi S, Ross A, Ma K, *et al*. Polymerase chain reaction screening for Y chromosome microdeletions: a first step towards the diagnosis of genetically-determined spermatogenic failure in men. *Mol Hum Reprod* 1996;2:775–9
71. Vogt PH, Edelmann A, Kirsch S, *et al*. Human Y chromosome azoospermia factors (AZF) mapped to different subregions in Yq11. *Hum Mol Genet* 1996;5: 933–43
72. Stuppia L, Gatta V, Calabrese G, *et al*. A quarter of men with idiopathic oligo-azoospermia display chromosomal abnormalities and microdeletions of different types in interval 6 of Yq11. *Hum Genet* 1998;102:566–70
73. Bonduelle M, Aytoz A, Van Assche E, *et al*. Incidence of chromosomal aberrations in children born after assisted reproduction through intracytoplasmic sperm injection. *Hum Reprod* 1998;13:781–2
74. Kurinczuk J, Bower C. Birth defects in infants conceived by intracytoplasmic sperm injection: an alternative interpretation. *Br Med J* 1997;315:1260–5
75. Mitchell AA. Intracytoplasmic sperm injection: offering hope for a term pregnancy and a healthy child? *Br Med J* 1997;315:1245–6
76. Bonduelle M, Wilikens A, Buysse A, *et al*. Prospective follow-up study of 877 children born after intracytoplasmic sperm injection (ICSI), with ejaculated epididymal and testicular spermatozoa and after replacement of cryopreserved embryos obtained after ICSI. *Hum Reprod* 1996;11(suppl 4):131–55
77. Loft A, Petersen K, Erb K, *et al*. A Danish national cohort of 730 infants born after intracytoplasmic sperm injection (ICSI) 1994–1997. *Hum Reprod* 1999;14:2143–8
78. Wennerholm UB, Bergh C, Hamberger L, *et al*. Incidence of congenital malformations in children born after ICSI. *Hum Reprod* 2000;15:944–8
79. Hewitson L, Simerly C, Schatten G. Cytoskeletal aspects of assisted fertilization. *Semin Reprod Med* 2000;18:151–9
80. Tesarik J, Sousa M. Comparison of Ca^{2+} responses in human oocytes fertilized by subzonal insemination and by intracytoplasmic sperm injection. *Fertil Steril* 1994; 62:1197–204
81. Aytoz A, Camus M, Tournaye H, *et al*. Outcome of pregnancies after intracytoplasmic sperm injection and the effect of sperm origin and quality on this outcome. *Fertil Steril* 1998;70:500–5
82. Luetjens CM, Payne C, Schatten G. Non-random chromosome positioning in human sperm and sex chromosome anomalies following intracytoplasmic sperm injection. *Lancet* 1999;353:1240
83. Bonduelle M, Devroey P, Liebaers I, van Steirteghem A. Major defects are overestimated. *Br Med J* 1997;315:1365
84. Bonduelle M, Joris H, Hofmans K, *et al*. Mental development of 201 ICSI children at 2 years of age. *Lancet* 1998;351:1553
85. Bowen JR, Gibson FL, Leslie GI, Saunders DM. Medical and developmental outcome at 1 year for children conceived by intracytoplasmic sperm injection. *Lancet* 1998;351:1529–34
86. Sutcliffe AG, Taylor B, Li J, *et al*. UK study of children born after intracytoplasmic sperm injection IVF: early report. Abstract 381. *Br J Obstet Gynaecol* 1998;105(suppl): 212–13
87. Bonduelle M, Liebaers I, Deketelaere V, *et al*. Neonatal data on a cohort of 2889 infants born after ICSI (1991–1999) and of 2995 infants born after IVF (1983–1999). *Hum Reprod* 2002;17:671–94
88. Ludwig M. Results of a German multicentre study to assess the efficacy and safety of ICSI. In Symposium Abstracts submitted to *Treatment Trends to Improve Success in Reproductive Medicine*. Lausanne, Switzerland: ESHRE, 2001

89. Laws-King A, Trounson A, Sathananthan H, Kola I. Fertilization of human oocytes by microinjection of a single spermatozoon under the zona pellucida. *Fertil Steril* 1987;48:637–42
90. Ng SC, Bongso A, Ratnam SS, *et al.* Pregnancy after transfer of sperm under zona. *Lancet* 1988;2(8614):790
91. Yovich JM, Edirisinghe WR, Cummins JM, Yovich JL. Influence of pentoxifylline in severe male factor infertility. *Fertil Steril* 1990;53:715–22
92. Yovich JL, Cummins JM, Morales P, *et al.* Pentoxifylline increases sperm penetration into zona-free hamster oocytes without increasing the acrosome reaction. *Andrologia* 1993;25:359–62
93. Hansen M, Kurinczuk J, Bower C, Webb S. The risk of major birth defects after intracytoplasmic sperm injection and in vitro fertilisation. *N Engl J Med* 2002; 346:725–30

5

Some newer developments in assisted reproductive therapies and their possible implications for children

'Plutus himself, that knows the tinct and multiplying medicine,
hath not in nature's mystery more science,
than I have in this ring'

William Shakespeare, *All's Well that Ends Well*, Act V, Scene III

Advances in assisted reproductive technologies (ART) occur continuously. These initially are at the basic science level often with animal work preceding the human studies. However, sometimes the preceding animal studies are few or simply do not exist. Studies that aim to investigate outcome are usually directed towards such things as pregnancy rates, implantation rates and other factors related to pregnancy. They seldom look at children born after these new variants of *in vitro* fertilization (IVF).

To illustrate this 'dive into the unknown' with lack of outcome work I will discuss the technique known as preimplantation genetic diagnosis (PGD). Two variants of this form of novel diagnostic technique were described by Handyside and colleagues[1] and Verlinsky and colleagues[2]. Both were developed directly using human embryos. In essence this technique involves removing one or two cells from an embryo conceived with IVF and intracytoplasmic sperm injection (ICSI) at the eight- to ten-cell stage of early human development (Figure 5.1).

When discussing an international outcome study to investigate the effect of PGD on early childhood growth and development, I visited centers in the USA, Australia and Europe. Whilst working with colleagues in a major

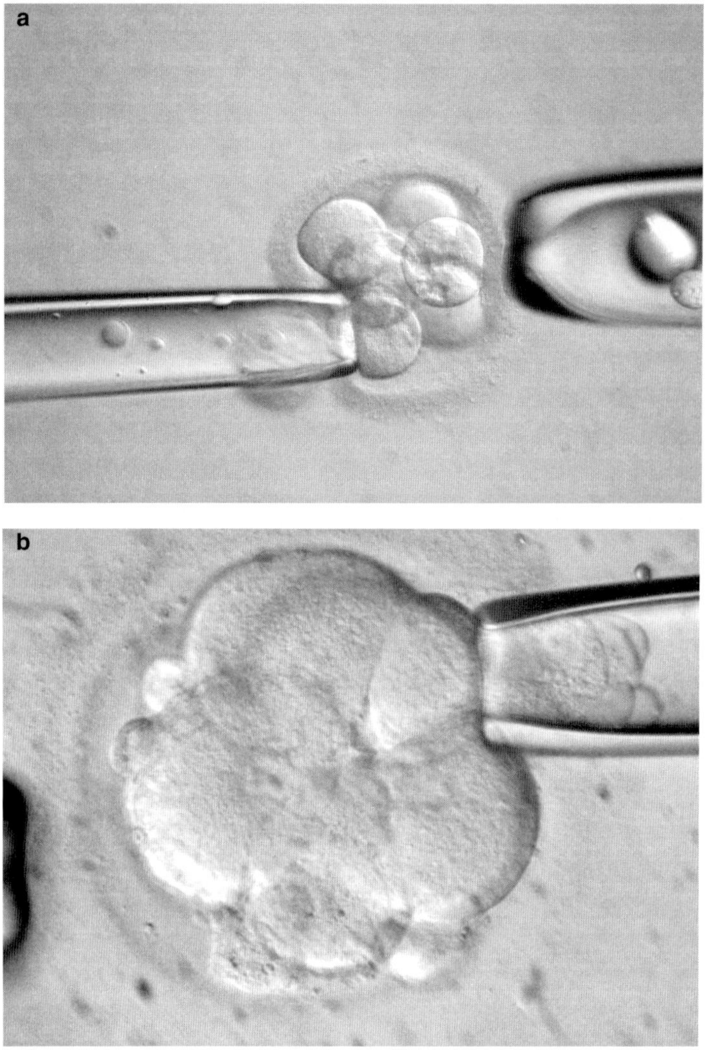

Figure 5.1 (a) Insertion of the needle into an embyo (created by *in vitro* fertilization) held in place by a micropipette; (b) withdrawal of one or two cells for preimplantation genetic diagnosis. Figures reproduced by kind permission of the Center of Reproductive Medicine, Dutch-Speaking Brussels Free University, Belgium

PGD center in the USA, I found that one of the pediatricians who had read my study design had discussed this new method with his wife, a musician. When she discovered that such a method existed, in which it is possible to reduce an embryo by up to 25% of its cell mass and then, if whichever condition for which it is being screened is excluded, that reduced embryo is placed into the mother, she was amazed that such a seemingly invasive method had not been subject to rigorous safety checks.

So far there has been only one outcome study looking at possible implications for babies beyond the neonatal period born post-PGD. This study[3] investigated the health of 109 infants with no control/comparison group. Data on perinatal outcome were gathered for their clinic's first 109 infants by parental reporting and confirmed by telephone interview and chart review when indicated. In infants > 6 months old, a follow-up telephone interview was performed establishing the developmental milestones attained by the child. So whatever data were obtained by that study, whilst laudable in its own way, would be of poor quality, unobjective and unlikely to show anything but the most gross problems.

PGD is performed at a very early stage of human development and adds to the complex mix of different factors that may have implications for children conceived after PGD. These factors need to include consideration that PGD is performed using IVF and is indeed available because of IVF. In most centers where PGD is performed, ICSI is also used. The reason for this is now discussed.

A typical family who may benefit from PGD would be one that had experienced the tragedy of loss of a previous child who had a lethal genetic disease. This allows the couple, when they conceive again, to be able to be screened for that particular disease. Therefore, it is imperative that the PGD technique be accurate. When testing biopsied blastomeres (i.e. cells taken from the blastocyst stage of embryonic development) it is imperative that any test is able to test the genome of that particular embryo. In PGD, however, because it is a technique that involves an *in vitro* fertilized egg (see Figure 1.2, page 9) the biopsy could by accident assay sperm DNA surrounding the fertilized egg. Therefore, ICSI is also used to be certain that only one spermatozoon is involved (unlike conventional IVF where an ovum is mixed with prepared sperm) and none surrounding the ovum (as in standard IVF) are potentially able to be biopsied by mistake. Thus PGD also exposes the future child to some of the risks of ICSI as well. The PGD technique thus gives an example of how increasingly complicated new methods have multiple potential risks for children conceived with their help.

PGD AS A RISK FACTOR

Let us now consider PGD alone and those risks that might be attributable to embryo biopsy *per se*.

PGD involves the embryo, which has already undergone IVF/ICSI, being exposed to an additional unknown risk. This risk arises from the exposure of the embryo to:

(1) Chemicals, such as acid tyrodes;
(2) Physical effects, such as laser, which is now used for zona drilling;
(3) The removal of one or two blastomeres at the six- to ten-cell stage of embryonic development;
(4) Direct damage from culture media secondary to zona drilling.

PGD is a novel diagnostic method used to investigate and prevent inherited diseases. Developed in the UK[1], its use is rapidly increasing in the early diagnostic testing of rare genetic diseases in high-risk populations (e.g. older mothers) and groups of families at risk. It is now used in an increasing number of fertility centers in Europe and throughout the world. Despite this increasing use, licensing bodies (e.g. the Human Fertilisation and Embryology Authority (HFEA), UK) have questioned the implications of this new technique for the health of children who were conceived after embryo biopsy, which involves a reduction of up to 25% of the cell mass of the developing embryo. Germany has banned this technique.

Since the first description of a successful human PGD pregnancy[1], the use of the technique has increased steadily, resulting in the birth of several hundred children worldwide[4,5]. In PGD the embryo is biopsied by removal of one or two cells (i.e. a reduction in embryo size of up to 25%), which are used for specific gene probing or fluorescent *in situ* hybridization (FISH) screening for chromosomal aneuploidy.

There is concern that reduced fetal size (which could be postulated to occur secondary to PGD) is associated with long-term health problems. The Barker hypothesis[6] suggests that several major diseases of later life, including coronary heart disease, hypertension and type 2 diabetes, originate from impaired intrauterine growth and development. These diseases may be consequences of 'programming', whereby a stimulus or insult at a critical, sensitive period of early life has permanent effects on structure, physiology and metabolism.

In an animal model Biggers and Papaioannou[7] examined the extent of postnatal compensatory growth in body weight and tail length of genetically identical F1 mice from three groups: the natural offspring of timed matings; transferred controls – offspring from embryos flushed at the two-cell stage and transferred to recipient foster mothers, and transferred half embryos – offspring developing from one blastomere from the two-cell stage transferred to recipient foster mothers. There was little difference between the postnatal growth curves of transferred controls and mice produced from half embryos, indicating that regulation during prenatal development is complete and that halving an embryo at the beginning of gestation has no lasting effects on its size or postnatal growth rate. In contrast, embryo transfer itself had a significant effect, resulting in smaller litters and larger, more variable animals after birth. There was then a period of postnatal compensatory growth in body weight and tail length after 4 weeks of age.

Hardy and colleagues, in an early study[8] of human preimplantation development *in vitro*, suggested that biopsy at the eight-cell stage was not harmful in humans. This in essence was a case study, reporting at birth and with no controls.

It is a salutary fact that, apart from reports from the European Society of Human Reproduction and Embryology (ESHRE), PGD special-interest group reports on outcome at birth in human pregnancies, there is only one report in the literature on PGD pediatric outcome[3].

Given the fact that PGD has so many potential applications, it is surprising that it has been used for so few families. This is partly due to the expense of the technique, but also because of concerns about its safety. ESHRE has established a voluntary registry in which details of the newborn babies (post-PGD) are recorded. However, such a registry system is reliant on voluntary informants and is therefore intrinsically flawed. Individual centers/groups do not have enough births to constitute a reliable case series or controlled study (allowing for power calculations) of outcome, and no large-scale collaborative controlled study has so far been initiated. It is from meetings held at ESHRE in June 2000 that it was decided to seek funding to undertake a robust scientific project looking beyond birth at children born post-PGD (Sutcliffe and associates, grant application for an international PGD outcome study; IPOS). IPOS will extend the work of the ESHRE voluntary registry[5,9], which has been responsible for the only consistent reporting on outcome after PGD.

In 1997 the ESHRE PGD consortium was formed as part of ESHRE's Special Interest Group on Reproductive Genetics, in order to undertake a long-term study of the efficacy and clinical outcome of PGD. This group provides only data at birth[5], but supports the IPOS proposal.

The ESHRE group's recent report[5] from 886 cycles (162 live-born children) summarizes the uses for this non-conventional diagnostic method as: genetic risk and objection to termination of pregnancy (TOP),

44.0%; genetic risk and previous TOP, 27.9%; genetic risk and sub- or infertility, 29.2%; age-related aneuploidy, 5.4%; others, 9%; noting that some cycles fit into several categories.

The rare genetic diseases that were diagnosed[5] using PGD at the time of the report included cystic fibrosis, thalassemia, spinal muscular atrophy (type 1,) Tay–Sachs disease, myotonic dystrophy, Huntington's chorea, Charcot–Marie–Tooth disease 1A, Duchenne/Becker's muscular dystrophy, fragile-X syndrome, hemophilia and Wiskott–Aldrich syndrome.

In the ESHRE report[5], 31 pregnancies were the subject of complications. There was a high number of couples with previously affected children (601 patients) and previous stillbirths (817 of the referred patients). Of the 162 live-born children[5] gender was skewed towards girls because of the high level of X-linked diseases. Apart from description of birth weight and maturity, little else was recorded about the children. Importantly, the ESHRE report[5] had no control group.

PGD is ever evolving with FISH for sexing, aneuploidy screening and structural chromosomal abnormalities[5], and fluorescent and multiplex polymerase chain reaction (PCR) as the most recent developments for monogenic diseases[5]. However, beyond birth, apart from the above-mentioned study[5], nothing is known about children post-PGD. It would be ironic if a technique developed to enable couples to have healthy children, of itself, harmed these children.

SKEWED X-CHROMOSOME INACTIVATION AND PGD

Here it is postulated that PGD may have another unexpected effect. In female mammals, dosage compensation for X-linked genes between XX females and XY males is achieved by transcriptional inactivation of genes on one of the two X chromosomes[10]. X-inactivation is mediated through a minimal region, the X-inactivation center (Xic), located in the human on Xq13, which is necessary for X-inactivation[11]. The *Xist/XIST* gene mapping to this region is expressed only from the inactive X-chromosome[12,13] and was demonstrated to be necessary to X-inactivation[14]. In the mouse, X-inactivation is first detected at the late morula/blastocyst stages of preimplantation development[15,16] and is restricted to the extraembryonic lineages in which the paternal X chromosome (X^P) is selectively inactivated[17,18].

Random inactivation of the maternal (X^M) or paternal (X^P) chromosome occurs later in the embryonic ectoderm lineage. Once a specific chromosome is inactivated (X^P or X^M), the same chromosome is kept inactivated through mitosis, and cells of clonal origin in general keep the same parental X inactivated. This process usually results in even inactivation of each X-chromosome in all adult tissues. In the human, very little is known about the initiation of the inactivation and there were contradictory results about the preferential inactivation of X^P in extraembryonic lineages[19,20].

In female adult tissues, each X-chromosome is generally found inactivated in an equal proportion of cells and it is expected that, at the time of the initiation of inactivation, a similar number of cells must inactivate the paternal and maternal X. By analogy with the mouse, we can postulate that the inactivation occurs randomly in the inner cell mass (ICM) or germ disk of female human embryos around day 7. The germ disk is then formed by at least 100 cells already differentiated into two sublineages: the epiblast and the hypoblast.

The mechanisms responsible for the initiation of inactivation lead to the inactivation in roughly an equal proportion of cells of the paternally inherited X-chromosomes (X^P) and maternally inherited X-chromosomes (X^M). These mechanisms are, up to now, completely unknown. Positional factors spreading evenly across the early embryo could be inducing the inactivation of one or the other chromosome. However, such a gross bipolar positional effect would probably not achieve even randomness in all derived tissues, as one could expect that cell clusters from the germ disk, precursors of different organs or tissues, would fall into one or the other zone of inactivation.

Alternatively, ICM cells could have inherited an imprint from an earlier generation of cells, even from the two- or four-cell stage, when a different imprint on each cell would guarantee a subsequent equal subdivision of the cells into X^P and X^M inactivated cells. This imprint would therefore precede the inactivation process and guarantee equal inactivation between the cells in all tissues derived from the embryo proper. In the trophectoderm cells, this 'random' imprint could be overruled by the parental imprint, which, in this lineage, might result in the X^P preferential inactivation.

For female patients heterozygous for an X-linked genetic disease, skewed inactivation has often been described, with positive or negative effects on the patient. For the mutations having a positive effect, it is thought that the mutant gene product induces a proliferative or survival disadvantage to the cells expressing it. In these cases the gene defect is at the origin of the skewing by negative selection against cells where the mutant X is active. This has been described in incontinencia pigmenti[21], Barth syndrome[22] and X-linked dyskeratosis congenita[23]. Most often, however, a skewed inactivation is detected in heterozygous females expressing a severe phenotype in a normally recessive condition. This has been described for numerous conditions, such as some mental retardation[24,25]; Duchenne muscular dystrophy[26]; ornithine transcarbamylase deficiency[27]; hemophilia B[28]; X-linked myotubular myopathies[29], Börjeson–Forssman–Lehmann syndrome[30]; Hunter's disease[31] and dystrophinopathies[32]. It is highly unlikely that a selective advantage could be gained through the presence of these single gene defects. It is more plausible that the skewed inactivation merely reflects what is found in the general population and is due to either a malfunction of the X-inactivation mechanism or the death of cells at a critical time, i.e. when it would induce a marked skewing. The severity of the skewing observed and the relatively high number of cases described in the literature indicate either an early predetermination of the X to be inactivated as postulated earlier, or a rather inaccurate and unreliable 'X-selecting' mechanism.

During PGD, one or two cells are removed for genetic analysis from, usually, an eight-cell stage embryo. Should, at that stage, one X already be marked for inactivation, the removal of two cells having the same imprinted chromosome could by itself initiate a strong inactivation bias. Furthermore, to avoid double piercing of the zona pellucida, adjacent blastomeres are usually biopsied and therefore are more likely to have the same imprinted X. For X-linked diseases, the biopsy, and other blastomere-damaging procedures such as embryo freezing, might increase the chances of skewed inactivation. For female children heterozygous for an X-linked recessive disease born following such a procedure, this would increase their risks of developing symptoms.

The irony of this phenomenon, if it proves to be real (due to be investigated by Ray, Bonduelle, Sutcliffe and others), is that if, for example, the family were being screened for Duchenne muscular dystrophy, then the very process of PGD may increase the risk that a female child thus born would have the condition PGD was supposed to be excluding! These are potentially murky waters into which we are being plunged. PGD serves as a very good example of the complexity of what may happen at the basic science level, let alone the child level.

RISK OF CANCER TO IVF-CONCEIVED CHILDREN

Earlier in the discussion above, reference was made to the Barker hypothesis. This states that a number of important adult diseases, including cardiovascular disease, hypertension and non-insulin-dependent diabetes, have their origin in fetal life[33]. A principle emerges from this, which is beautifully simple: changes to an individual in early life can make lasting changes to them in adulthood. There is a substantial body of evidence derived from animal work to support this hypothesis, but no absolute mechanism of action has been discovered ... yet. The mechanism by which the Barker hypothesis is manifested at the cellular level is bound to be complex and multifactorial. This mechanism is the source of intense scientific enquiry, with one promising area being consideration of the relevance of 'genomic imprinting'.

A little about genomic imprinting

The phenomenon of genomic imprinting was discovered in the early 1980s by two independent pieces of research. One group was performing a comprehensive genetic analysis of translocations in the mouse genome and discovered that specific regions of the genome produced reproducible phenotypes when one parental region was deleted or duplicated, but no effect when the other parental region was affected[34]. This was the first indication of non-equivalence of the two parental copies of specific genes. This work also showed that genes that were imprinted were not randomly distributed throughout the genome but more closely located on particular chromosomes. Another group[35] used micromanipulation to create mouse embryos with either two female or two male pronuclei. The 'female' embryos had larger placentae and smaller fetuses while the 'male' embryos had normal placentae and larger fetuses. None survived until term. After the phenomenon was discovered, a number of distinctive syndromes and cancers have been identified in humans that arise as a result of abnormal genomic imprinting (Table 5.1).

Genomic imprinting and its possible implications for IVF conception

Imprinting is a dynamic process, informing the chromatin structure to mediate monoallelic expression (imprint formation), and manifesting monoallelic expression throughout life. Imprinted genes may be particularly vulnerable to disruption, as they are functionally haploid and their expression is regulated by different means from the rest of the genome. Since imprinted genes are functionally haploid, they may be more vulnerable to inducing disease states when subjected to mutations or epimutations.

Table 5.1 Candidate conditions arising as the result of gene imprinting

Condition	*Major features*	*Frequency in population**
Prader–Willi syndrome	babies are born floppy, with characteristic facial appearance; they have low IQ and hyperphagia	1 in 16 000
Angelman's syndrome	so-called 'happy puppet' syndrome; unable to speak, severely delayed development with characteristic appearance	1 in 30 000
Beckwith–Weidemann syndrome	neonatal hypoglycemia and overgrowth of the tongue, pancreas and generalized overgrowth; long-term risk of Wilms' tumor	1 in 14 600
Russell–Silver syndrome	a form of asymmetrical dwarfism with pseudohydrocephalic appearance	sporadic
Wilms' tumor	kidney tumor developing in mid-childhood; can be cured if diagnosed early	9.8/100 000
Osteosarcoma	bone cancer (5% of child cancer); can be cured, but often results in disability	6.8/100 000
Bilateral retinoblastoma	neonatal eye tumor which can cause blindness, but if detected early can be cured without any loss of vision	3.8/100 000
Rhabdomyosarcoma	very serious embryonic tumor of the muscle; rarely cured	4.7/100 000

*All very rare. Any risk from IVF conception is not quantified and may be non-existent

These mutations are more likely to occur in an abnormal environment such as *in vitro* (although every effort has been made to make the IVF media as physiological as possible).

As stated above, a number of rare diseases have been discovered to manifest due to genomic imprinting, which is now considered to be an epigenetic phenomeon. It has been suggested that the epigenetic phenomenon involved in genomic imprinting may be influenced by IVF. A survey (Sutcliffe, Peters and participant IVF units in the UK) will attempt to find evidence for or against this hypothesis, by enquiring about the occurrence of known rare conditions, throughout the UK, in children who have been conceived by IVF. To date, around 50 text-imprinted genes have been identified (See http://www.mgu.har.mrc.ac.uk/imprinting/imprinviewdatagenes.html). Many have not been fully cloned or still have unknown function. This survey will be aimed at those syndromes/diseases that have a known, defined phenotype and would be likely to be familiar to parents who had a child affected by one of them.

If this survey reveals any evidence for higher rates of occurrence of the defined conditions below, further studies will need to be initiated, to investigate imprinting as a possible secondary feature of IVF. The syndromes and cancers that are already known to be caused by genes which are imprinted include: Prader–Willi syndrome, Angleman's syndrome, Russell–Silver syndrome and Beckwith–Weidemann syndrome; the cancers are bilateral retinoblastoma, Wilms' tumor, osteosarcoma and rhabdomyosarcoma. A summary of their features and incidences are in Table 5.1. It must be noted that these conditions are all rare, fortunately, but this of course means that if there was a mechanism then it would be difficult to recognize.

Interestingly, the very first IVF-conceived child I saw who had been conceived after replacement of a frozen embryo[36] had Beckwith–Wiedemann syndrome as a baby. At the time, I had said to myself after seeing the child that I had found the cause for Beckwith–Wiedemann syndrome. Little did I know that, owing to advances in knowledge since then, this naive remark may have been closer to the truth than I thought!

OTHER ADVANCES IN ART

There are continuing innovations in the ways of treating infertile couples, which may or may not constitute additional risk to the children born. This chapter concludes with descriptions of these.

Hormonal regimes and IVF children

So far, detailed consideration has not been given to the changes in ovulation regimes that are used to achieve ovulation in an IVF cycle. Here, it is believed that the primary risks are to the mother and not the child. However, lessons learnt from the use of diethylstilbestrol are worth mentioning when considering whether there is evidence that hormones given to expectant mothers could have risks for children born after ART. Whilst diethylstilbestrol was not involved in IVF treatment protocols, previous experience with that hormone reminds us that caution is still necessary when using new unknown hormones (e.g. gonadotropin releasing hormone (GnRH) anatagonists) in new IVF protocols.

To summarize briefly, diethylstilbestrol was used extensively in America to prevent early abortions. These were not IVF pregnancies. Later, when daughters born to mothers treated with stilbestrol were growing up, a very rare tumor of the vagina started to appear in teenage daughters of these mothers. The administration of diethylstilbestrol to women during pregnancy was associated with an increased risk of vaginal or cervical adenocarcinoma in their exposed female offspring[37]. The link between this tumor and its use during their mother's early pregnancy was then discovered ... too late and with tragic consequences.

New hormonal regimes such as the use of GnRH anatagonists are continuously being introduced. These may have implications for children, but there are fortunately no other specific examples where hormonal use during IVF regimes has been directly linked to fetal or child anomalies 'post-stilbestrol'.

Blastocyst transfers

Another area of change is in delaying the replacement of embryos after conventional IVF. In order to improve embryo quality, there is currently an effort to maintain the embryo for 48 h in the *in vitro* environment. This method allows the embryo to grow into a more mature embryo called a blastocyst (see Figure 3.2, page 41). The hope is that the weaker embryos will not continue to mature and those ultimately viable for transfer will be of 'higher quality'. Again, this may hold extra risks for any child conceived this way. An example of such a risk is the increased possibility of monozygotic twinning. It has been long recognized that higher-order births are more common after IVF (this is referred to in other chapters), but it has also been observed that there is also curiously a higher rate of monozygotic twinning after IVF.

Monozygotic twinning and IVF

This topic has been more thoroughly reviewed in *Iatrogenic Multiple Pregnancy*[38]. However, it is worthy of brief commentary here, since in this chapter two of the techniques specifically implicated in the etiology of monozygotic (MZ) twinning (blastocyst transfer and PGD) have been discussed.

From early in the history of IVF[39] a rise in the rate of MZ twinning was noted. It had been suggested even before ART[40] that a rise in the rate of MZ twinning occurred after the introduction of the oral contraceptive pill. There is more recently emerging evidence that blastocyst transfers, and indeed any method that involves zona drilling/manipulation of the

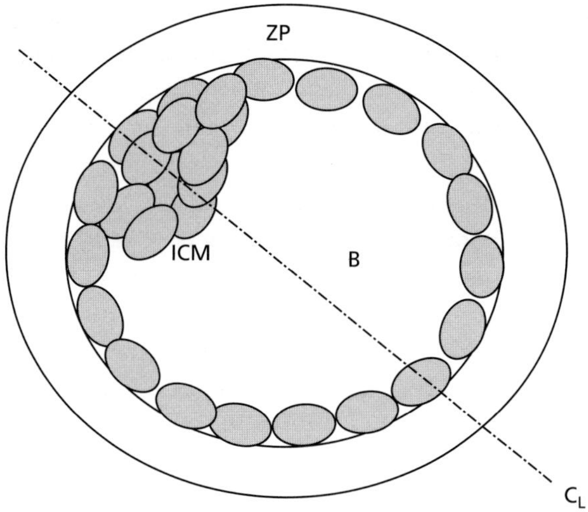

Figure 5.2 Diagram of blastocyst (about 200 cells) depicting the relationship of the zona pellucida (ZP), the blastocele (B) and the inner cell mass (ICM). Mechanical splitting of an embryo has produced monozygotic twins in laboratory animals, and deformation subsequent to blastocyst passage through an artificial zona opening has been proposed to yield similar results. A cleavage plane (C_L) bisecting this early conceptus favors complete duplication of the embryo and development of monozygotic–dichorionic twins. Figure reproduced with permission from Sills ES, Tucker MJ, Palermo GD. Assisted reproductive technologies and monozygous twins: implications for future study and clinical practice. *Twin Res* 2000;3:217–23

embryo, may result in a higher risk of MZ twinning. Factors implicated in the process include:

(1) Impaired hatching caused by prolonged embryo culture; this disturbs the zona pellucida;
(2) Manipulation of the zona pellucida (using laser or acid tyrode);
(3) The use of supraphysiological ovulation-induction agents (should artificial induction of ovulation harden the zona pellucida unevenly, any weakness would result in potential herniation).

The zona pellucida

Early work recognized the zona pellucida 'the ovule itself is found to consist of an external membrane, the zona pellucida'[41], and its importance is now recognized in fertility. The functions of this structure are now being increasingly elucidated (Figure 5.2). Amongst others, these include a species-specific polyspermy barrier. The importance of the zona pellucida is reflected in the fact that there is only one recorded case of its absence, and this woman was infertile[41]. The zona pellucida limits blastocyst contact with the endometrium and therefore became a target for therapeutic intervention. Zona drilling was one of these interventions. This is an attempt to overcome perceived difficulties with the zona by weakening it to allow sperm access to the oocyte by use of laser or acid tyrodes.

Results from animal experiments suggest that MZ twinning can be induced from zona pellucida manipulation (e.g. zona drilling). Manipulation of the zona necessarily occurs in PGD, as discussed earlier. It has been assumed but never observed that the process of zona manipulation for whatever purpose could be the cause of the observed increased rates of MZ twinning in ART pregnancies and births.

Other evidence concerning the mechanisms underlying MZ twinning comes from animal studies. These studies suggest that a change in the timing of developmental events could contribute to this process. Stockard[42] induced MZ twinning in fish by reducing O_2 supply or temperature to interrupt certain cleavage stages. Delayed ovulation as a possible mechanism has been seen in several animal species. Vincristine given to mice at day 7 of pregnancy induces MZ twinning in the baby mice. Massip and Van der Zwalmen[43] observed herniation of a cow blastocyst through a hole in the zona pellucida. This division into two halves resulted in two ICMs (see Figure 5.2). This process has never occurred in a human embryo to completed pregnancy, but has been observed in an embryo replaced, which did not go to term. It should be added that the scientific community is unsure whether blastocyst transfer or zona pellucida manipulation are the cause of MZ twinning after ART; interested readers can review the current literature[44–51].

Evidence that there is an increased rate of MZ twinning post-ART

Pharaoh and colleagues[52], examining HFEA figures, have found that there are a large number of unaccounted for same-sex twin pairs after ART in relation to what may be predicted from birth registry data. From the East Flanders twin survey[53] it is possible to estimate the rate of zygote splitting from rates of singleton and other births this is reported as 0.7% and 0.2 times that of spontaneous ovulation. Other groups studying IVF pregnancies have estimated varying rates of MZ twinning from 0.61 to 2.4%, all above the expected norms[38]. Assisted hatching of the human blastocyst in its various forms has been observed to be associated with a higher rate of MZ twinning[54].

Why is a rise in monozygotic twinning more important than dizygotic twinning?

The topic of twinning and its importance in IVF has been discussed in detail in Chapter 4. No specific mention of difficulties that arise uniquely to MZ (identical) twins has been made so far. This is a large topic, but worthy of summary comment here.

Most difficulties arise in MZ twins during pregnancy, as a result of a condition called twin–twin transfusion syndrome (TTTS). In this condition there is abnormal exchange of blood between the twins, who are in essence linked to the same placenta (unlike dizygotic twins, where each twin has a different placental system). The effect of the single placental system when TTTS arises is that one twin becomes a net donor of blood and the other becomes a net recipient of blood (via aberrant blood vessels in the common placental system). The donor twin becomes anemic, hypoxic and growth-restricted and the recipient twin becomes edematous and goes into catastrophic heart failure. The edematous twin constantly attempts to excrete the extra fluid (blood) it is inadvertently receiving from its co-twin. This is produced as fetal urine. This fluid dramatically increases the maternal amniotic fluid volume, resulting in premature labor. Untreated severe cases have 100% mortality. Almost all MZ twin pregnancies have some degree of this process going on.

Treatments are available, but even after treatment there is major morbidity from this disease process. Severe TTTS occurs in about 15% of monochorionic twin pregnancies and, untreated, is associated with a high mortality[55,56]. Several treatments have been introduced to try to improve pregnancy outcome, including selective feticide, cord ligation and repeated amniodrainage[57–59]. More recently, fetoscopic laser ablation of the intercommunicating vessels has been described[60], resulting in 70% of pregnancies with at least one survivor[61] and possible reduction in serious morbidity such as cerebral palsy, compared to the initial experience with amniodrainage[62].

In the study by Sutcliffe and co-workers[63] examining outcome after laser ablation therapy for TTTS, there was no cerebral palsy in the singleton survivors but there were five cases in the twin group (a rate of 9%). All except one affected child (with quadriplegia) had mean Griffiths scores in the normal range. However, study numbers were small, and this finding must be considered in the context of the very poor outcome with untreated severe TTTS, the uncertain outcome following alternative therapies and the unknown long-term outcome in unselected monochorionic twin pregnancies. No study to date has examined the development of such cohorts (apart from that of Minakami and co-workers[64] discussed below). From the study of Sutcliffe and associates and others it is obvious that any process associated with increased MZ twinning is one to be introduced with caution in view of the known higher morbidity from MZ twinning (e.g. markedly higher rates of cerebral palsy).

Other risks of monozygotic (monochorionic) twin pregnancies

It has long been recognized that cerebral palsy is more common in twin pregnancies, with the main associated risk factors being preterm birth, low birth weight and intrauterine growth restriction[64]. In the Western Australian 1980–89 birth registry study of cerebral palsy, of 5132 twins, 38 were found to have cerebral palsy, but this study was unable to assess the effects of chorionicity[65]. In a study of the effects of chorionicity on infant outcome at 1 year, Minakami and co-workers[64] showed, in a study of 44 monochorionic and 164 dichorionic twin pregnancies, that adverse outcomes such as death, cerebral palsy and mental retardation occurred in 10% of the monochorionic infants but only 3.7% of the dichorionic infants and in their study TTTS was judged to have affected 32% of the monochorionic pregnancies. Pharoah and Adi[52], in a recent retrospective survey of survivors of *in utero* death in a co-twin, found an overall risk of cerebral impairment of 20% in the survivor. Finally, in a perinatal outcome study from the Australian–New Zealand Twin–Twin Transfusion Syndrome Registry[66], where amniodrainage was used as the treatment for 82.1% of cases, an abnormal cranial ultrasonographic scan was noted in 27.3% of live-born neonates. The risk of death or significant morbidity following the death of a co-twin in monochorionic twin pregnancies is about 25%[67,68]. In the study of Sutcliffe and colleagues[63], the singleton survivors appeared to be of normal ability and there were no cases of cerebral palsy in this group, supporting the hypothesis that laser ablation therapy protects the survivor in the event of an *in utero* co-twin death. Morbidity and mortality following *in utero* co-twin death in monochorionic twin pregnancies is a consequence of the development of hypotensive episodes secondary to the presence of flow through the vascular anastomoses. Doppler studies have demonstrated reversed blood flow from the live fetus to the dead twin immediately following *in utero* death of the co-twin. Fetal blood sampling after death demonstrates anemia in the surviving fetus, and ultrasonographically visible cerebral lesions may subsequently develop in the survivor in the following weeks[67,69]. The aim of systematic coagulation of all superficial placental vessels that cross or are adjacent to the intertwin amniotic membrane is to interrupt the vascular communications between the circulations of the two fetuses. Although arteriovenous anastomoses (which are thought to play the major role in the hemodynamic disturbance underlying fetofetal transfusion) are found deep in common cotyledons, their afferent and efferent branches are superficial, and coagulation of all crossing vessels will inevitably include the supply to these anastomoses. Recent attempts at selective ablation of a small number of arteriovenous anastomoses under direct vision may potentially reduce the risk of possible procedure-related co-twin death secondary to severe uteroplacental insufficiency. However, since some anastomoses, especially arterial–arterial, may remain, the observed 'protective' effect of ablation of all crossing vessels may be attenuated. The outcomes of studies reporting such selective procedures are awaited.

The study of Sutcliffe and colleagues[63] again highlighted a need in this case, when performing an invasive treatment for high-risk conditions in pregnancy, for adequate detailed developmental follow-up of the children born, to assess long-term well-being and morbidity.

In vitro maturation

The world's press were ebullient about the announcement in 1999 that a woman who had ovarian tissue removed, frozen and later replaced into her body appeared to have recovered ovarian function[70]. Typically there was a gross overinterpretation of the ramifications of this case report, with the unrealistic expectation that children and young adults who have to have chemotherapy and total body irradiation may later recover their fertility by having their germline tissues frozen before treatment and replaced later. This assumes that any primordial germ cells taken from a sexually immature prepubescent child may mature 'naturally' if returned to their body later. Whilst the self-healing properties of the human body never fail to impress those dedicated to the care of sick children, the quantum leap in knowledge required to achieve this renders such speculation naive.

However, other scientists for different reasons are using a different strategy to try to advance treatment. So-called *in vitro* maturation involves the harvest of immature oocytes followed by their maturation in an *in vitro* environment to the point where they would normally be released in an ovulatory cycle (typically day 14).

Gosden[71] has shown that it is possible to mature a day 7-harvested ovum to 'day 14 of the cycle' *in vitro*. An egg matured in this manner is much more likely to fertilize, implant and develop into a normal pregnancy (although this has not been attempted to date) in relation to one that is released under hormonal superstimulation. This has the potential to obviate the necessity to use artificial gonadotropin-stimulated cycles to release ova of less certain maturity. By avoiding hormonally stimulated polyovulation this may solve a fundamental problem of present IVF treatment, namely the birth of twins, triplets and other higher-order births. This is a single mature oocyte that is likely to be fertilized and produce a single embryo, which can be placed in the expectant mother with the knowledge that it is likely to develop into a mature pregnancy. This technique of *in vitro* maturation has no child outcome data, because it is too new.

Oocyte cryopreservation

Cryopreservation of oocytes is a technique developed to preserve oocytes of patients undergoing cancer treatment or for oocyte donors. Cryopreserved oocytes require ICSI for fertilization (after thawing) because the cryopreservation process brings about changes in the zona pellucida preventing sperm penetration[67]. Only cryopreservation of mature oocytes has been successful. Following this has been the first report of successful cryopreservation of mature ovarian tissue and reimplantation into the same patient 10 years later (referred to above[70]).

This has led to speculation about the possibility of cryopreservation and subsequent *in vitro* maturation of immature germ cells. This is of unknown risk. A mouse named Eggbert has been born after the first successful maturation from a primordial germ cell. Eggbert died young and was obese, diabetic and had developed intestinal lymphosarcoma[69]. Does any more need to be said to convince the reader to be cautious when considering that new reproductive technologies are safe for children?

CONCLUSIONS

Developments in ART continue apace; some of these have been discussed in this chapter. However, the outcome studies needed to monitor these have not all been performed. Careful thought needs to go into this area of protocol development, as can be seen by the above discussion, which highlights a variety of ways in which risks arise. These can be from such differing mechanisms as gene imprinting, embryo biopsy, increased rates of MZ twinning, risk of skewing of X^M/X^P inactivation and other factors. These have to be considered over and above those risks (fortunately few on the basis of known outcome) that arise from standard IVF and/or ICSI.

REFERENCES

1. Handyside AH, Kontogianni EH, Hardy K, Winston RML. Pregnancies from biopsied human preimplantantion embryos sexed by Y-specific DNA amplification. *Nature (London)* 1990;344:768–70
2. Verlinsky Y, Ginsberg N, Lifchez A, *et al.* Analysis of the first polar body: preconception genetic diagnosis. *Hum Reprod* 1990;5:826–9
3. Strom CM, Levin R, Strom S, *et al.* Neonatal outcome of preimplantation genetic diagnosis by polar body removal: the first 109 infants. *Pediatrics* 2000;106:650–3
4. Palermo G, Joris H, Devroey P, Van Steirteghem AC. Pregnancies after intracytoplasmic injection of single spermatozoon into an oocyte. *Lancet* 1992;340:17–18
5. Geraedts J, Handyside A, Harper J, *et al.* European Society of Human Reproduction and Embryology Preimplantation Genetic Diagnosis Consortium Steering Committee ESHRE preimplantation genetic diagnosis (PGD) consortium: data collection II (May 2000). *Hum Reprod* 2000;15:2673–83
6. Barker DJ, Hales CN, Fall CH, *et al.* Type 2 (non-insulin-dependent) diabetes mellitus, hypertension and hyperlipidaemia (syndrome X): relation to reduced fetal growth. *Diabetologia* 1993;36:62–7
7. Biggers JD, Papaioannou VE. Postnatal compensatory growth of manipulated mouse embryos. *Hum Reprod* 1991;6:36–44
8. Hardy K, Martin KL, Leese HJ, *et al.* Human preimplantation development *in vitro* is not adversely affected by biopsy at the 8-cell stage. *Hum Reprod* 1990;5:708–14
9. Geraedts J, Handyside A, Harper J, *et al.* ESHRE Preimplantation Genetic Diagnosis (PGD) Consortium: preliminary assessment of data from January 1997 to September 1998. ESHRE PGD Consortium Steering Committee. *Hum Reprod* 1999;14:3138–48
10. Lyon MF. Gene action in the X-chromosome of the mouse (*Mus musculus* L.). *Nature (London)* 1961;190:372–3
11. Brown CJ, Lafreniere RG, Powers VE, *et al.* Localization of the X inactivation centre on the human X chromosome in Xq13. *Nature (London)* 1991;349:82–4
12. Brown CJ, Ballabio A, Rupert JL, *et al.* A gene from the region of the human X inactivation centre is expressed exclusively from the inactive X chromosome. *Nature (London)* 1991;349:38–44
13. Brockdorff N, Ashworth A, Kay GF, *et al.* Conservation of position and exclusive expression of mouse Xist from the inactive X chromosome. *Nature (London)* 1991; 351:329–31
14. Penny GD, Kay GF, Sheardown SA, *et al.* Requirement for Xist in X chromosome inactivation. *Nature (London)* 1996;379:131–7
15. Epstein CJ, Smith S, Travis B, Tucker G. Both X chromosomes function before visible X-chromosome inactivation in female mouse embryos. *Nature (London)* 1978; 274:500–3

16. Monk M, Harper MI. Sequential X chromosome inactivation coupled with cellular differentiation in early mouse embryos *Nature (London)* 1979;281:311–13
17. Takagi N, Sasaki M. Preferential inactivation of the paternally derived X chromosome in the extraembryonic membranes of the mouse. *Nature (London)* 1975;256:640–2
18. West JD, Frels WI, Chapman VM, Papaioannou VE. Preferential expression of the maternally derived X chromosome in the mouse yolk sac. *Cell* 1977;12:873–82
19. Migeon BR, Do TT. In search of non-random X inactivation: studies of fetal membranes heterozygous for glucose-6-phosphate dehydrogenase. *Am J Hum Genet* 1979;31:581–5
20. Goto T, Wright E, Monk M. Paternal X-chromosome inactivation in human trophoblastic cells. *Mol Hum Reprod* 1997;3:77–80
21. Smahi A, Courtois G, Vabres P, *et al.* Genomic rearrangement in NEMO impairs NF-kappaB activation and is a cause of incontinentia pigmenti. The International Incontinentia Pigmenti (IP) Consortium. *Nature (London)* 2000;405:466–72
22. Orstavik KH, Orstavik RE, Naumova AK, *et al.* X chromosome inactivation in carriers of Barth syndrome. *Am J Hum Genet* 1998;63:1457–63
23. Vulliamy TJ, Knight SW, Dokal I, Mason PJ. Skewed X-inactivation in carriers of X-linked dyskeratosis congenita. *Blood* 1997;90:2213–16
24. Raynaud M, Moizard MP, Dessay B, *et al.* Systematic analysis of X-inactivation in 19XLMR families: extremely skewed profiles in carriers in three families. *Eur J Hum Genet* 2000;8:253–8
25. Lossi AM, Millan JM, Villard L, *et al.* Mutation of the XNP/ATR-X gene in a family with severe mental retardation, spastic paraplegia and skewed pattern of X inactivation: demonstration that the mutation is involved in the inactivation bias. *Am J Hum Genet* 1999;65:558–62
26. Yoshioka M, Yorifuji T, Mituyoshi I. Skewed X inactivation in manifesting carriers of Duchenne muscular dystrophy. *Clin Genet* 1998;53:102–7
27. Yorifuji T, Muroi J, Uematsu A, *et al.* X-inactivation pattern in the liver of a manifesting female with ornithine transcarbamylase (OTC) deficiency. *Clin Genet* 1998; 54:349–53
28. Chan V, Chan VW, Yip B, *et al.* Hemophilia B in a female carrier due to skewed inactivation of the normal X-chromosome. *Am J Hematol* 1998;58:72–6
29. Tanner SM, Orstavik KH, Kristiansen M, *et al.* Skewed X-inactivation in a manifesting carrier of X-linked myotubular myopathy and in her non-manifesting carrier mother. *Hum Genet* 1999;104:249–53
30. Kubota T, Oga S, Ohashi H, *et al.* Borjeson–Forssman– Lehmann syndrome in a woman with skewed X-chromosome inactivation. *Am J Med Genet* 1999;87:258–61
31. Sukegawa K, Song XQ, Masuno M, *et al.* Hunter disease in a girl caused by R468Q mutation in the iduronate-2-sulfatase gene and skewed inactivation of the X chromosome carrying the normal allele. *Hum Mutat* 1997;10:361–7
32. Azofeifa J, Voit T, Hubner C, Cremer M. X-chromosome methylation in manifesting and healthy carriers of dystrophinopathies: concordance of activation ratios among first degree female relatives and skewed inactivation as cause of the affected phenotypes. *Hum Genet* 1995;96:167 76
33. Barker DJ. *In utero* programming of chronic disease. *Clin Sci (Lond)* 1998;95: 115–28
34. Cattanach BM, Kirk M. Differential activity of maternally and paternally derived chromosome regions in mice. *Nature (London)* 1985;315:496–8
35. Surani MA, Sasaki H, Ferguson-Smith AC, *et al.* The inheritance of germline specific epigenetic modifications during development. *Philos Trans R Soc Lond B Biol Sci* 1993;339:165–72

36. Sutcliffe AG, D'Souza SW, Cadman J, *et al.* Minor congenital anomalies, major congenital malformations and development in children conceived from cryopreserved embryos. *Hum Reprod* 1995;10:3332–7
37. Herbst AL, Ulfelder H, Poskanzer DC. Adenocarcinoma of the vagina. Association of maternal stilbestrol therapy with tumor appearance in young women. *N Engl J Med* 1971;284:878–81
38. Blickstein I, Keith LG, eds. *Iatrogenic Multiple Pregnancy: Clinical Implications*. London: UK: Parthenon Publishing, 2001
39. McDonagh PG. Discussion of Mason C Andrews, *et al.* An analysis of the obstetric outcome of 125 consecutive pregnancies conceived *in vitro* and resulting in 100 deliveries. *Am J Obstet Gynecol* 1986;154:848–54
40. Bressers WM, Eriksson AW, Kostense PJ, Parisi P. Increasing trend in the monozygotic twinning rate. *Acta Genet Med Gemellol (Roma)* 1987;36:397–408
41. Jones HW Jr. Foreword. In Veeck LL. *Atlas of the Human Oocyte and Early Conceptus*. Baltimore: Williams and Wilkins, 1986:vii
42. Stockard CR. Developmental rate and structural expression: an experimental study of twins, 'double monsters' and single deformities, and the interaction among embryonic organs during their origin and development. *Am J Anat* 1921;27: 115–262
43. Massip A, Van der Zwalmen P. Atypical hatching of a cow blastocyst leading to separation of complete twin half blastocyst. *Vet Rec* 1983;112:301
44. Schachter M, Raziel A, Friedler S, *et al.* Monozygotic twinning after assisted reproductive techniques: a phenomenon independent of micromanipulation. *Hum Reprod* 2001;16:1264–9
45. da Costa AL, Abdelmassih S, de Oliveira FG, *et al.* Monozygotic twins and transfer at the blastocyst stage after ICSI. *Hum Reprod* 2001;16:333–6
46. Behr B, Fisch JD, Racowsky C, *et al.* Blastocyst-ET and monozygotic twinning. *J Assist Reprod Genet* 2000;17:349–51
47. Schieve LA, Meikle SF, Peterson HB, *et al.* Does assisted hatching pose a risk for monozygotic twinning in pregnancies conceived through *in vitro* fertilization? *Fertil Steril* 2000;74:288–94
48. Sills ES, Moomjy M, Zaninovic N, *et al.* Human zona pellucida micromanipulation and monozygotic twinning frequency after IVF. *Hum Reprod* 2000;15:890–5
49. Hershlag A, Paine T, Cooper GW, *et al.* Monozygotic twinning associated with mechanical assisted hatching. *Fertil Steril* 1999;71:144–6
50. Meldrum DR, Wisot A, Yee B, *et al.* Assisted hatching reduces the age-related decline in IVF outcome in women younger than age 43 without increasing miscarriage or monozygotic twinning. *J Assist Reprod Genet* 1998;15:418–21
51. Alikani M, Noyes N, Cohen J, Rosenwaks Z. Monozygotic twinning in the human is associated with the zone pellucida architecture. *Hum Reprod* 1994;9:1318–21
52. Pharaoh PO, Adi Y. Consequences of *in-utero* death in a twin pregnancy. *Lancet* 2000;355:1597–602
53. Loos R, Derom C, Vlietinck R, Derom R. The East Flanders Prospective Twin Survey (Belgium): a population-based register. *Twin Res* 1998;1:167–75
54. Cohen J, Talansky BE, Malter H, *et al.* Microsurgical fertilization and teratozoospermia. *Hum Reprod* 1991;6:118–23
55. Sebire NJ, Snijders RJM, Hughes K, *et al.* The hidden mortality of monochorionic twin pregnancies. *Br J Obstet Gynaecol* 1997;104:1203–7
56. Saunders NJ, Snijders RJM, Nicolaides KH. Therapeutic amniocentesis in twin–twin transfusion syndrome appearing in the second trimester of pregnancy. *Am J Obstet Gynecol* 1992;166:820–4

57. Dommergues M, Mandelbrot L, Delezoide AL, *et al.* Twin-to-twin transfusion syndrome: selective fetocide by embolisation of the hydropic fetus. *Fetal Diagn Ther* 1995;10:26–31
58. Lemery DJ, Vanilieferinghen P, Gasq M, *et al.* Fetal umbilical cord ligation under ultrasound guidance. *Ultrasound Obstet Gynecol* 1994;4:399–401
59. Mahony B, Petty C, Nyberg D, *et al.* The stuck twin phenomenon: ultrasonographic findings, pregnancy outcome and management with serial amniocentesis. *Am J Obstet Gynecol* 1990;163:1513–22
60. Ville Y, Hyett J, Hecher K, Nicolaides K. Preliminary experience with endoscopic laser surgery for severe twin twin transfusion syndrome. *N Engl J Med* 1995;332: 224–47
61. Ville Y, Gagnon A, Sebire NJ, *et al.* Endoscopic laser coagulation in the management of severe twin-to-twin transfusion syndrome. *Br J Obstet Gynaecol* 1998;105: 446–53
62. Nicolaides DH, Hyett J, Ville Y, Hecher K. Management of severe twin-to-twin transfusion syndrome and twin reversed arterial perfusion sequence. In: Ward RH, Whittle MJ, eds. *Multiple Pregnancy.* London: RCOG Press, 1995:251–62
63. Sutcliffe AG, Sebire NJ, Taylor B, Edwards PR, Nicolaides KH. Outcome for children born after *in-utero* ablation therapy for severe twin-to-twin transfusion syndrome. *Br J Obstet Gynaecol* 2001;108:1–5
64. Minakami H, Honma Y, Matsubara S, *et al.* Effects of placental chorionicity on outcome in twin pregnancies. A cohort study. *J Reprod Med* 1999;44:595–600
65. Petterson B, Nelson KB, Watson L, Stanley F. Twins, triplets, and cerebral palsy in births in Western Australia in the 1980s. *Br Med J* 1993;307:1239–43
66. Dickinson JE, Evans SF. Obstetric and perinatal outcomes from the Australian and New Zealand twin–twin transfusion syndrome registry. *Am J Obstet Gynecol* 2000; 182:706–12
67. Murphy KW. Intrauterine death in a twin: implications for the survivor. In Ward RH, Whittle M, eds. *Multiple Pregnancy. London: RCOG Press,* 1995:218–30
68. Nicolini U, Poblete A. Single intrauterine death in monochorionic twin pregnancies. *Ultrasound Obstet Gynecol* 1999;14:297–301
69. Jou HJ, Ng KY, Teng RJ, Hsieh FJ. Doppler sonographic detection of reverse twin–twin transfusion after intrauterine death of the donor. *J Ultrasound Med* 1993; 12:307–9
70. Radford J, Shalet S, Lieberman B. Fertility after treatment for cancer. Questions remain over ways of preserving ovarian and testicular tissue. *Br Med J* 1999; 319:935–6
71. Gosden RG. Survival of transferred C57BL mouse embryos: effects of age of donor and recipient. *Fertil Steril* 1974;25:348–51

6

Some concluding thoughts

'To be, or not to be: that is the question'.

William Shakespeare, *Hamlet*, Act III, Scene I

In its broadest context, the term 'infertility' includes both subfertility and absolute sterility. Biologically it implies that the capacity to produce offspring is diminished; statistically it is observed as a decrease in the actual number of children produced. The subject of human infertility is complex and is not fully understood by those who receive treatment for it, those who provide these treatments (which are rapidly expanding) and those who care for the children thus conceived.

In the UK there have been over 30 000 children conceived via *in vitro* fertilization (IVF) and the first child born following IVF will be 24 years old on 25th July 2002. Recently introduced techniques have resulted in increased pregnancy and live birth rates, and in the case of intracytoplasmic sperm injection (ICSI) have resulted in a new group of couples being able to have their own child without resort to adoption or artificial donor insemination. In Europe alone by 1999 there were 100 000 ICSI-born children.

These children represent a significant group and will want to know in the future if they have been conceived in this way. Regrettably it is not the intention of every parent to inform them. Even in Sweden, where the law was changed to make availability of identifying data for sperm donors compulsory, parents in this particular type of assisted reproduction are still reticent to tell their children. In my present European study of 5-year-old ICSI-conceived children, the UK part has already assessed more than 300 IVF children. It is clear to us that, although we are advising all families to tell their children at a young age about their mode of conception, some are opting not to. This is in part due to a lack of appropriately worded/orientated literature to inform such discussions, but more importantly some parents have taken the unwise decision never to tell their children about their mode of conception. The fact that only 20% of the Swedish families[1] had told their children about donor sperm comes as no surprise. I accept that these families are a special case and likely to be much more secretive than other ART families, but in my opinion this does give us some idea of what is happening in the more general context of assisted reproduction.

The 'first generation' will, when mature, come to represent a powerful client group whose questions concerning how they were conceived are likely to be far reaching. Ideally we should anticipate some of their questions when new treatments are being introduced and advocated. No one involved in fertility treatments will be immune from blame should the nightmare scenario arise of assisted reproductive technologies (ART) having long-term deleterious consequences (e.g. higher risks of cancer or neurological disease). It may be with the increasing power of patient advocacy groups and increasing regulation of all things medical that there will be a day when outcome studies on new reproductive therapies become mandatory. Some ethics committees are taking the responsible decision, with new therapies (ICSI is one case that has been identified), to insist on mandatory follow-up. Prospective and informed consideration of these issues with carefully designed studies to investigate risks should be established immediately in areas where they have not been already.

Costs of these studies need to be taken into consideration at the start of the introduction of novel ART therapies. Those who perform them should ideally have neither a constituency nor funding from any part of the process of ART, neither from the large number of innovative companies who fund and develop new treatments nor from the clinics that perform these treatments.

The issue of outcome of course touches on one of the many ethical considerations concerning the use of ART. Where does the responsibility of those involved in the treatments end and what responsibility do they have to children born after these treatments?

On balance, the evidence in this book concerning children born after IVF (and its variants) suggests that, when born mature and singleton, these children are no worse off than their naturally conceived peers. The only caveat is that there is a slightly increased background risk of congenital anomalies in relation to naturally conceived children and they are slightly lighter at birth[2]. In the case of ICSI, the risks of congenital anomalies seem to be similar, but where a Y-chromosome microdeletion exists, with present techniques this will be passed on to male children. A remaining issue, the fertility of males born after ICSI, will be revealed only when these boys grow up.

In the case of premature birth and children from higher-order births, IVF children are exposed to the same risks that naturally conceived children are, and there are now methods being adopted to reduce this risk, such as reducing the numbers of embryos replaced per IVF cycle. It is hoped that in the future risks of having triplets or more will further decrease.

Whilst we may be optimistic about the future for IVF children, despite some of the concerns raised in Chapter 5, too many steps too soon can have disastrous consequences. In a mouse model, scientists under supervision of John Eppig developed a mouse (Eggbert) from a primordial germ cell. Eggbert died young and was obese, diabetic and had developed intestinal lymphosarcoma. Critically these problems developed after full physical maturity was attained[3].

Whilst evidence to date suggests that IVF-conceived children are healthy, it is unsafe to draw any conclusions about their long-term well-being. Caution needs to be exercised when considering the implications for potential children whose parents have conceived with help from these new reproductive technologies. Whilst infertility has sometimes devastating effects on an individual's sense of completeness and self-worth, the health of the child should be paramount in further developments of these new techniques. These children bring joy to their parents and their interests should be at the center of any consideration of new or indeed existing fertility methods. A nation's children are its investment in the future.

FINALLY

This book has discussed a wide range of available knowledge pertinent to understanding where IVF children are from and where they are going, including aspects of genetics, andrology, gynecology, obstetrics, teratogenesis, neurodevelopmental pediatrics, epidemiology, neonatology and other subjects. A subject that has been largely avoided is medical ethics and its relevance to the use of new untested technologies.

From readings of articles discussing ethical issues with ART, a eugenic slide can be perceived. Subjects considered and elegantly argued to be off limits are now argued sometimes by the same individuals to be safe, ethical and necessary. We are on the brink of attempts being made to clone human beings and here again the ethicists are against ... but no, some are drawing parallels with 'nature's clones' monozygotic twins. One might cynically believe that it will not be long before those generating arguments will arrive at one that justifies cloning. These advocates rarely seem to act in the interests of the child.

The introduction of this book started with some consideration of extracorporeal conceptions according to Greek mythology, and with Greek mythology it will thus end.

Pandora was the first woman on earth. Zeus ordered Hephaestus, the god of craftsmanship, to create her and he did, using water and earth. The gods endowed her with many talents; Aphrodite gave her beauty, Apollo music, Hermes persuasion, and so forth – hence her name: Pandora, 'all-gifted'.

When Prometheus stole fire from heaven, Zeus took vengeance by presenting Pandora to Prometheus' brother. With her, Pandora had a jar, which she was not to open under any circumstance. Impelled by her natural curiosity, Pandora opened the jar, and all evil contained escaped and spread over the earth. She hastened to close the lid, but the whole contents of the jar had escaped, except for one thing which lay at the bottom, and that was Hope. Let us hope that:

(1) Those who develop these new technologies respect the sanctity of human life;
(2) Those who benefit from them by being able to conceive will continue to do so;
(3) Those children born from these treatments will not be exposed to risks as the result of a failure to consider the ethical as well as the technical aspects of introducing new technologies;
(4) The further development of such treatments is not leading to an opening of Pandora's jar.

REFERENCES

1. Gottlieb C, Lalos O, Lindblad F. Disclosure of donor insemination to the child: the impact of Swedish legislation on couples' attitudes. *Hum Reprod* 2000;15:2052–6
2. Schieve LA, Meikle SF, Ferre C, *et al*. Low and very low birth weight in infants conceived with use of assisted reproductive technology. *N Engl J Med* 2002;346:731–7
3. Eppig JJ, O'Brien MJ. Comparison of preimplantation developmental competence after mouse oocyte growth and development *in vitro* and *in vivo*. *Theriogneology* 1998;49:415–22

Index